# HEAL
*your*
# HOME 2
*The Next Level*

*Also by Adrian Incledon-Webber*

### Books

Heal Your Home

Spirit & Earth (Co-authored with Tim Walter)

### DVD

Intuition – Your Hidden Treasure

(available as a download)

### Courses

The Secrets of Healing Your Home I, II and III

Introduction to Dowsing
Dowsing for Health I and II
Earth Energies I
Healing with Sacred Symbols
Spirit & Earth I, II and III

### Online Store

www.dowsingspirits.co.uk

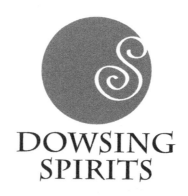

# DOWSING SPIRITS

# HEAL *your* HOME 2

## *The Next Level*

The mistakes and experiences from our past make us who we are today, but they don't need to define who we might become, or what we can achieve in the future.

As channelled to Adrian, 2nd January 2021

# Acknowledgements

This book is dedicated to Allyson and Annie, both of whom have been my constant companions on this journey. One has kindly kept me supplied with toast, whilst the other helped eat it.

I could not have completed any of my books without them by my side, or in Annie's case, by my feet. Thank you from the bottom of my heart.

To my boys Alistair and Charles, each year I have grown more proud of them. Two hard working, honest men that I am honoured to call my sons and best friends.

To Jess, a very welcome addition to the I-W's, I could not have wished for a better daughter in law.

And to Natalie, I hope that you make an honest man of him soon.

James McNeill and Mark Ames, a very big thank you for lending me the Coach House for two weeks, it allowed me to really crack on with the book, couldn't have done it without you. The gin and tonics kept me going!

Lottie and Tracy, two very special friends, it means a lot to me that you are there.

My fabulous and talented editor Michelle, without whom the books (all three of them) would probably never have made it to print. A very big thank you.

And Huw, the amazing guy that has done all the artwork for my books, DVD, logos etc. He has never failed to come up with the goods, so intuitive and insightful.

Sukhi and Malkit. Their beautiful home in Crete where *Heal Your Home 2* started. I admit that it was not easy to leave the sunny patio and start typing but I hope that the end result makes you proud.

And, of course, to all the people who bought *Heal Your Home* and my clients worldwide, thank you all for your support. The wonderful feedback received from you over the last few years encouraged me to write this sequel.

To all my dowsing mates out there, you know who you are.

I was told by a Medium some years back that I would write at least four books. I am not sure what the next one will be, but keep an eye open.

# Contents

# Editor's Note

When I met Adrian's wife, Allyson in 2012, I had no idea that my casual offer to advise her husband on how to get his book published would result in him becoming my client of 8 years, with three books completed, or that we would also become friends in the process. Eight years ago, Adrian trusted me with helping to publish his book, *Heal Your Home*, and it has since helped many people, myself included, to clear and heal themselves and their homes of detrimental energies.

The world is shifting and changing more rapidly now than ever before, and it is so important that we not only recognise lower energies that need healing or releasing, but that we are able to release them and heal them for ourselves. When I first read *Heal Your Home*, back in 2013, what struck me was that out of all the dowsing and healing books I had read (having been dowsing since 2005) it was the only one that actually offered actionable, concrete solutions to the issues. It was not simply telling you how to find the problems, it was also telling you how to fix them, and that, to me, was pure gold. Especially as none of the solutions required fancy ingredients or tools or skills that the average person does not have.

Working with Adrian on his books is always a pleasure, not only because they are books on topics that I am passionate about, and am thrilled to be able to help create, but also because Adrian is devoted to helping others to live their lives unencumbered by negative energies and influences, and so is willing to work hard to make the books as easy to read and to use as possible. This new edition has taken on a slightly different format to the first, and we hope that it is even easier to use, and that healing your home and your life is simpler than ever, because you deserve to live your life joyfully, without external forces negatively affecting you.

Michelle Gordon

Author of *Where's My F\*\*king Unicorn?*
and the *Earth Angel Series*
February 2021

# Introduction

It is often said that as soon as a book is published it is out of date, and I didn't want that to be the case for my first book, *Heal Your Home*, or the courses that I teach. As a result, the information in *Heal Your Home* is very much 'evergreen', but over the last seven years since it was published, there have been many new discoveries, which have prompted me to write this edition.

As planetary energies change, so do we. Our thoughts, our beliefs and of course, our healing methods are ever-evolving. Nothing stays the same and that is the reason for this new book.

I have never been one to stand still. I am always looking for and willing to accept guidance from above. Each house and family that I work on is an education, another step toward further honing the skills that I have been given. I will always be eternally grateful to my friend and mentor Andy Roberts for speaking the immortal words 'You too can do this' in the midst of a healing session. It set me off on a path that I could not even have imagined.

Thanks to *Heal Your Home*, I have connected with amazing and wonderful people from all over the world and the feedback has been outstanding. People are reading my book, taking on board what I have written and then are using the healing methods that I have given them. This fulfils the main purpose for me writing the first book, to empower people to help and heal themselves. This new edition, *Heal Your Home 2*, will also enable you to carry out additional healing on your own home and family, taking it to the next level.

Writing these books is rather like giving people a rod and teaching them to fish rather than just giving them food. That way they can help themselves rather than relying on others to provide what they need. When I hear about readers beginning to individualise how they carry out the healing, I am thrilled. I have also been told on many occasions that as soon as my book enters a home, the healing process begins. The book itself seems to have taken on a life force of its own, which is something that I never expected or imagined.

Some of the new information I have to share, has been channelled and some of it has come from the need to delve further into a problem faced by clients during the healing work on their homes and family.

When working on a house it is rather like a detective novel, you never know what you are going to find, rarely do you know where it is going to lead, and finally what new discoveries you might make along the way.

It is dealing with these new discoveries that has brought about these new additions to my checklist. It may never be a finalised list. Increased sensitivities, with mobile phones becoming more powerful, and being hit by intensive EMF's and microwaves from Smart Meters etc., will cause the list to grow. And of course, the healing will need to change and develop with it.

Seven years ago, my editor and I decided to leave a number of chapters out of *Heal Your Home*, mainly on E.T.s (or Off-Worlders, as I prefer to call them,) to ensure the creditability of the book. Most of what I wrote about in *Heal Your Home* was totally new information to many people; and my editor, Michelle, didn't want me to include any chapters or information that might alienate (no pun intended) or destroy any credence or confidence that people would have in the book, and I had to agree with her thoughts. But now, in *Heal Your Home 2*, we can let rip!

There are now fifty-six questions to work through. Some of the titles of what to look for have been slightly changed from *Heal Your Home* mostly to bring them up to date with my current thinking, and some of the topics are brand new.

Although the book is called 'Heal Your Home', I would say that probably 60% of the healing is done on the people within the home. Our homes contain many noxious energies, but so do humans. A client once said to me 'The family is so much healthier and happier since you healed our house'. Working on the family and clearing away the inherent emotional problems that we all face, helps enormously. It gives us an inner strength that we all perhaps had but lost somewhere along the way.

Life is hard and we can easily get worn down mentally, physically, and spiritually by the stresses and strains of modern living, and the joy of life gets eroded. Recent world events including the virus outbreak have further compounded these issues, as fear and worry have pervaded our daily lives, making life even more difficult.

We are all on the money-go-round, and we often forget to have fun. In fact, I would say that we don't know what fun is anymore, as the days roll into weeks, then months and finally years before we perhaps see a flicker of light at the end of the tunnel. The light that the Dalai Lama would now call 'liberation' (aka enlightenment). This is the realisation that your life is not what it should be, and you then begin to change your whole outlook. You become a seeker, trying to find the answer to those elusive questions that have agonised people for years: 'Why are we here?' and 'What is my life all about?'.

By clearing ourselves of the emotional baggage that we carry, especially parental programming, we stand a chance of moving forward, to see life as it truly is and then start to help others.

My gift to you is this book, which holds the tools to start your journey.

Adrian Incledon-Webber
Richmond, Yorkshire
February 2021

# Part One

*Reasons to Dowse and Heal your Home*

# Why should you heal your home?

We need to become responsible for ourselves, and for our own wellbeing. And by buying this book and following the methods to heal your home and your family and yourself, this is exactly what you are doing. I want to touch upon some of the ways in which detrimental energies in your home can affect your life, and the lives of your loved ones, and how important it is that you take your time to work through this book.

I highly recommend that you set aside time on a regular basis to check that your home and family are clear of detrimental energies. I like to check my own home once a week, just to ensure nothing has become attached to a family member, or the shifting energies haven't produced any detrimental energies that weren't there before.

Sean O'Geary, a very old friend of mine, once said to me 'Before you can become Self-Less, you have to become Self-ish'. I remember being both confused and annoyed at the same time. I think that I was somewhere in my late 20s and hadn't had the life experiences that would eventually lead me to knowing what Sean meant and then fully agreeing with his statement.

So, what did Sean mean? Let's take plumbers as an example, (or electricians, decorators, or in fact any tradespeople). They spend all their time working on other people's homes and businesses making sure that they are safe, they have running water, heat etc. But more often than not, their own homes are in need of work, perhaps one radiator doesn't work, or the kitchen tap leaks… there is always something to be done, but they are so busy working on other people's houses that they rarely have time for their own.

Exactly the same happens within the healing world. So many healers spend too much time working on other people, and not enough time meditating, healing, and taking good care of themselves. So, the best thing you can do for your own health, and for the benefit of your family, is to ensure that you are completely clear of all and any detrimental energy patterns. The simplest way to do this, is to use the psychic protection method each morning and also to work through this book.

I believe it is imperative that all healers work on themselves before they start to work on others. By giving yourself healing each day you are not being selfish, you are being sensible and in the long run, more giving and selfless. We all need good foundations beneath our feet, to be fully grounded, it gives us a solid base which helps us not only use the healing power of Mother Earth but also to channel the white light from above.

Meditation is always said to play a key role in leading a spiritual life, to be able to calm the mind and body, to release all thought, all tension, all worries, all stress and just BE. Even after years of healing practice, I still find that very difficult to do, because as soon as I close my eyes to meditate, an individual name or family comes into my head for healing. Should I, as you are taught to do, clear away that thought and keep going with my meditation or should I stop and carry out the necessary healing work?

A conundrum indeed.

In most cases, the healing work wins, and the meditation goes completely out the window, so much for stilling the mind. I do try and maintain a balance, but with the sort of work that I now do, people come first and me second. But I do ensure, with the help from Mother Earth and the Universe, that my energies are replenished, so that my own health and wellbeing do not suffer in helping others to heal.

# Health and Wellbeing

If there are noxious energies in our homes or attachments connected to our auras, it will most certainly have a detrimental effect on our health and wellbeing. Often, the issues that arise can confound doctors and medical tests, because they are energetic, and therefore undetectable by blood tests and scans.

Often, we can feel the effects of these energies before they have made a physical impact on our bodies. If we can clear and harmonise the energies within our homes, often these aches and pains will disappear before they can have a tangible effect on our bodies that if left could possibly require medical intervention.

This is why it is so important for you to take responsibility for your health and the health of your family and not to expect an overworked doctor, who may only have 10 minutes to fully diagnose your problems and then prescribe the right treatment, to remedy all of your physical and mental issues.

If you work diligently through this book, carrying out a healing on anything that is affecting you detrimentally, it can help to restore the body's natural balance (homeostasis). Helping your mind and body to be at ease with themselves can often allow their natural healing ability to be restored.

**This book is not intended to replace mainstream medicine, there is a place for both in this world. If you are worried about your condition or illness, or that of your family, please do seek medical advice as soon as you can.**

As well as healing the energetic problems addressed in this book, keeping a food diary could help you ascertain whether there are any particular foods or drinks that may be causing you health problems. If you see any patterns, relating food to your symptoms, you can start to eliminate them from your diet to see if your symptoms begin to improve. Although medical doctors are now beginning to take nutrition into account, they often do not have the necessary time to spend on individual cases, so you may find it worth your while, if you think that food intolerances may be the problem, to seek out a good naturopath or nutritionist.

Taking responsibility for your health means carrying out research into the medications that you or a family member have been prescribed as some can have serious side effects, especially when taken with other drugs. I am always surprised at the cocktail of drugs people take, and then comment as to how unwell they feel after taking them. But they still keep taking them.

Many people still see their doctor as an authority figure and follow what they say to the letter. But no matter how good their intentions are, you are only one that truly knows your own body, and it is therefore imperative that you become your own health detective.

If you feel that you are suffering from side effects of any of the drugs that you are taking, ask your doctor to review them, as another pharmaceutical company may be manufacturing one that is more compatible with you.

My mother came from a generation that held the medical profession in such high esteem that she would take or do anything they told her to. My father was the same, his dining room table was full of bottles or packets of tablets that he had to take each day. I once asked him what they were for and he said, 'That one is for my heart, that one is to help thin my blood, that one is a statin, this is for my diabetes' and so it went on, he would take most of them twice a day.

In his late 70s, my father lost all sense of taste and smell due to the medications he was taking. He passed away shortly after his 84th birthday and he hadn't enjoyed his food for years. He even stopped drinking beer, and if you had known him you would realise how significant that was. A glass of his favourite Scotch was still a favourite tipple, but I wasn't sure how much he tasted it or if he just enjoyed the memories that it brought back.

All the pills and potions he was taking had their individual side effects, it said so on the leaflets inside the packets. But it didn't tell you what side effects may occur when taking all six or seven pills together.

I asked him one day why he took them all, and his answer was 'because the doctor told me to'. It took me back to my early teenage years when coming home from school one day with a report slip from the Headmaster saying that I had got into trouble doing something out of character. My father asked me why I did it, and my answer was 'because so and so told me to'.

His response was 'If I told you to put your head in a bucket of water for ten minutes, would you do it?' Obviously, I said no. 'Well then don't do what other people tell you to do, don't follow the herd'. Great advice.

So, I used exactly the same words on him, forty years later, regarding the pills he was taking. But his answer was 'You're not the one who is ill, I am'. I said that wasn't a constructive answer and asked again why he taking all the pills, and his answer this time was 'The doctors know best, don't they'.

He had given away the complete responsibility for his health to another human being. Knowing the Doctor's Surgery, I am sure that they were doing what they felt was best for my father, but they don't know everything there is to know when it comes to the side effects of taking multiple tablets.

None of this is said to diminish the need for mainstream medical practices, as there have been some remarkable breakthroughs over the centuries with the eradication of many diseases and improved treatments for illnesses and injuries. But what I am trying to say is that we can all do so much more to help ourselves on a daily basis, by taking more responsibility for our own health and wellbeing, rather than expecting someone else to fix us. I feel that dowsing is the perfect tool to enable you to do just that. You can use it to diagnose and to heal.

To repeat what my friend Sean said, all those years ago, 'Before you can become Self-Less you have to become Self-ish'. So, make sure you spend time, every day, looking after yourself, before you start to take care of everyone else.

# Dementia

Cases of dementia and Alzheimer's seem to be on the rise and many families have had loved ones affected by these awful, cruel, and debilitating illnesses. I wanted to write about this as it is one that is close to my heart as my father, who passed away some years back, was diagnosed with dementia.

My Ma had passed away some 10 years before, and though he quickly settled into a life by himself, we noticed that he was becoming a little forgetful, not overly so, but more than usual. In the beginning we didn't take too much notice, putting it down to his advancing years, until one day he collapsed.

Luckily, he didn't hurt himself, physically, but it did shake him up mentally and he seemed to go downhill very quickly after that. Before this happened, he had bought himself an apartment in Cambridgeshire to be near my brother, as I was still moving around and was never sure where I would end up living. Sadly, he never ended up moving into the apartment, as his dementia suddenly took a turn for the worse and it just wasn't safe for him to live alone any longer.

My brother found a very good nursing home near to where he lived, and they catered for people in all stages of dementia. Its proximity meant that Perry could go and visit Boy (as we called him) every day. I will always be grateful to him for taking on this responsibility, as it is not easy to see a loved one slipping away, day by day.

As his dementia worsened, I worked on him each day keeping him clear of attachments and any other detrimental energies that might be around him. I would also work on keeping the nursing home cleared of any spirits, any human manifested forms and all detrimental earth energies that might affect him and the other residents, as appropriate.

When I went to see him, I would always do some grounding work, making sure he was attached to Mother Earth. I had discovered earlier that Boy was not always present in his own body, his mind was often elsewhere, and this seems to be common amongst dementia and Alzheimer's sufferers. Therefore, to enable me to have a conversation with Boy, I needed to ensure that he was anchored to the planet, for him to be fully present in his physical body.

When visiting him I would always say that I was off to 'Planet Inky' (his other nickname was Inky) as I never really knew what I would find when I got there or how lucid he would be. He would often see things in his room that I couldn't, however I was quite prepared to believe that they were there, as I feel that dementia may well allow us to dip into another dimension.

In fact, during one visit, he mentioned seeing black blobs in the garden, so I quietly did some healing, asking for them to be cleared, soon after, he commented that they had gone. So, I feel that when in these altered states, those with dementia may be more open to glimpsing the unseen world and even possibly entering parallel worlds.

This become apparent when Allyson and I went off to see Carol Green, a talented medium, who was holding a clairvoyant evening in Cheltenham. Towards the end of the evening, she looked at me and said, 'Your Father is here'. I was a little surprised as Carol is normally in contact with the dead, those who have passed over who wish to contact their living relatives. But Boy was still alive at this point. I didn't reply to her comment, and she followed up with 'I know that he is still with us, but he is spending much of his time in the spirit world, has he got dementia?' I replied that, yes, he was still with us and that he had dementia.

She then said, 'He is spending this time in the spirit world as they are trying to convince him that there is, indeed, life after death, your mother is also spending time with him, which will ease his passing'. She continued 'He is with us for a while yet, but as he passes you will know, from his face, that he finally has realised he is going to an amazing place and that your mother was there to help move him through'. This was interesting considering he was not a spiritual person, and as far as he was concerned, once you passed over that was it. Life had no real meaning, you were born, you lived, then you died.

About 10 months later I received the call from Perry, to say that I had better get over to the nursing home as Boy wasn't looking too good and that he was slipping away. It took me two hours to drive there, and by the time I arrived he had gone, I had missed his passing by 15 minutes. Now, I have not seen many dead people in my life, so I was not fully prepared for what I saw when I walked into his room. His physical body was still laying on the bed, with a blanket pulled up to his chin, but the best description of what I felt was 'The lights were off, and no one was home'. There was no glow, there was what I can only describe as a husk on the bed, his spirit or soul had definitely flown.

I sat quietly for a few minutes, taking it all in. I was not tearful, as I knew he had been taken care of, and now the pain had gone. As I walked out of the room a nurse stopped me and said 'I was with him when he passed over, I was holding his hand, and suddenly, he opened his eyes, looked up and a beautiful smile suddenly appeared on his face. It was like he recognised someone hovering above his bed. The next minute, he was gone'.

That was exactly what Carol had said would happen and I admit at that moment I lost it, and tears fell from my eyes. Not from sadness, but at the thought that my mother was there for him and the beauty of his passing moment.

Dementia is a cruel disease, taking your loved ones away mentally and also physically. In many cases they become unrecognisable from the person they once were. But I do believe that their internal struggle can be eased by you carrying out a daily clearing of all the detrimental energy patterns surrounding them, and any attachments, by using the psychic protection method, and this can be sent, by you, from a distance. Grounding will certainly help them too, especially if they are constantly visiting other dimensions.

14

# Energy Work

I have had many people, who used my first book to carry out a healing on their homes, tell me that their energy work improved after doing so. Reiki practitioners, healers, and alternative therapists have found that their practices benefited from clearing their own homes/healing rooms of detrimental energies, and then protecting themselves and making sure that they were not picking up any attachments from their clients as they worked on them. They also started to incorporate many of the healing methods described in part four of the book, within their own healing practices, further helping their clients.

It's true that if you asked the average person on the street what Reiki was some 30 years ago you may well have received a blank stare and a shrug of their shoulders. But there are now thousands of practitioners worldwide bringing help and relief to millions of people both young and old alike. Even if they have never experienced it themselves, most people have now heard of these alternative healing methods, as well as many other associated complementary therapies.

So why the sudden rise in popularity?

I feel that it is because many people are wanting to take control of their own health and that of their family's too, seeking something, anything, that they can do to bring beneficial changes to their lives. It is not just the spiritual connection that attracts people to Reiki, or even the ability to set up a business from their home whilst bringing up a family, but a real compunction to make a change, to look at life in a different way. There's a desire to bring a positivity into their homes which in turn will bring a harmony to their lives that had been missing before.

At the beginning of my healing journey, when I was still running my Estate Agency business (Burns and Webber), I was having regular healing sessions with Andy Roberts. It was during one of these sessions that he suggested that I become attuned to Reiki, and therefore, on a sunny afternoon in Ash Vale, I went through my initiation ceremony for Reiki Level 1 and I remember feeling very calm as Andy carried out the ritual, implanting the various symbols into my aura.

During my drive home, which was about 45 minutes, I felt quite floaty, and that something had changed within me. Little did I know what was going to happen next. I had read several books on the subject before I became attuned, and thought I knew everything about the '21-day cleansing period' that followed. I was prepared for the possible headaches, the changing energies in my body and mind, the sleepless nights and vivid dreams, but I wasn't prepared for the feeling that I was getting during the last 15 minutes of my drive home.

Let's just say that it involved a very quick trip to the toilet. Luckily, I had a downstairs cloakroom in my house as I would not have made it upstairs. I called Andy to ask if this was normal and all I got was hysterical laughter from the other end of the telephone. So much for healing energy. I must say I was not convinced at that point.

Of course, everyone reacts very differently to these attunements, and many people, including my wife Allyson, don't suffer any kind of detrimental reaction at all. It is a very personal process.

After my attunement, I moved rapidly into the spiritual world of healing. I was not just on the receiving end but also able to help others. To me it was a whole new ball game.

At that time, going from my Estate Agency business to becoming a healer felt like a very natural progression. But others around me were not convinced. I can see that it must have seemed very strange, one minute a successful businessman and the next a healer. But I was off flying, reading books on as many subjects as I could. Andy helped direct me at this time, suggesting Drunvalo Melcheizadek's *Flower of Life* books, Hamish Miller and Paul Broadhurst's *Sun and the Serpent* and Sandy Stephenson's *The Time is Right*.

My interest in the healing realms was a way of taking responsibility for my own health, and I would certainly encourage anyone to explore any form of spiritual healing, whether Reiki or other alternative therapies that may resonate with them.

To me, healing is an essential by-product of spirituality, I don't think that you can start to live a more spiritual way of life without healing becoming a natural part of what you do. You become more aware of nature and how we affect the planet. By switching to a greener household cleaning product, for instance, means that you are helping, in some small way, to heal the earth.

What really interested me in Reiki was the ability, in Reiki Level 3, to send absent or distant healing to people all over the world. I could not get my head around the concept to begin with as it seemed so vast and I felt overwhelmed by what it could mean to everyone on the planet. It was incredible to me that anyone, no matter where they lived, could share in the healing that Andy had bestowed on me via Reiki.

Imagine seeing a photograph of someone who is in distress and being able to help them in some small way by just pausing for a few moments and sending a healing thought to them. Isn't that amazing and unbelievable all at the same time?

After many years of developing my healing practice, I don't tend to use Reiki anymore, but it has been a wonderful stepping stone and I would urge anyone starting out on their spiritual adventure to include this form of healing in their toolbox. It starts with self-healing and then moves rapidly onwards to include many other valuable lessons that will change yours and other people's lives for the better.

Although Reiki is still part of me, and the symbols are still there, I would now refer to what I do as 'Universal Healing'. I combine many different forms of healing when working on people and their homes, including some of the new solutions that I have been given from Upstairs (the

Universe) whilst trying to puzzle out how to rid a house of a new energy pattern that I have just found.

It is best to take baby steps when you start out on this wonderful and enlightening pathway, however, Upstairs have a habit of accelerating your journey. Start with healing yourself first, this will help strengthen and prepare you as you reach the first of many crossroads that you will come across along the way.

# Self-Love and Self-Esteem

If you are being affected by detrimental energies in your home, have a spirit or attachments within your aura, or a psychic cord tied to you, the chances are, your self-esteem and self-worth may be affected. These energies can contribute to making you feel low, worthless, and even unlovable.

Then if you have been raised by parents who were also adversely affected by these detrimental energy patterns, that will have a knock-on effect, also contributing to how good or bad you feel about yourself.

Sometimes, when teaching a course, I throw out, to the attendees, the following question: 'How much do you love yourself on a scale of 1 to 10?' I rarely get anyone saying 10 out of 10. Anything less than 10 actually means that you don't love yourself. How can it? If you love yourself then the answer has to be 10, nothing less.

It is possible to get to a point where you can completely love and accept yourself, your whole self: mind, body and spirit; but it is a lot easier to do so without any external energies affecting you detrimentally. Once they are cleared, harmonised, and healed, you will be able to work on self-love and acceptance, stepping into your true power, to be who you really are.

By picking up this book, and working through the diagnostic and healing sections, you are starting to empower yourself, giving yourself the ability to create the life you wish to lead, to be who you want to be.

There is no one else like you anywhere, as even in a parallel life you would be slightly different. You are the sum total of a unique upbringing, no one else has had the same experiences as you. We all have had to deal with hardships, we suffer from different types of abuse and bullying, working through many trials and tribulations as we go through life, but no one will have seen what you have seen.

You are a unique, talented, special, beautiful spark of divine light. And I hope that the process of working through this book will be just the beginning of your journey to loving yourself and seeing yourself in that light.

Start by giving yourself a huge pat on the back as you have come a long way since being born. Look at what you have learned over the years, look at the people you have influenced and helped over that time, the love that you have experienced and given to others, the insights and knowledge you have passed on. Every person that you meet will take a part of you with them and, of course, you never know when you interact with someone what beneficial influence they will have on you and you on them.

And remember, self-love is not selfish. It is building a solid foundation from which you can be of even more service to others.

# Parental Patterning

I would guess that for many people the problem of self-love, or lack of it, goes back to childhood. And as I mentioned earlier, that could well be because our parents have been affected by the detrimental energies that they have come into contact with during their lives. These repeating patterns can emerge especially when properties are passed down through the generations, you can see children having the same issues as their parents and even their grandparents before them.

If you inherit a property from family, it is best to carry out a full house healing, cutting any ties to the past, especially if there was an illness involved in their passing. Any strife, over the years, within the family unit will also need to be cleared away and a healing carried out. Even the mildest argument can leave a detrimental trace behind that can affect you years later.

Parents cannot teach their children what they do not know or understand themselves, and so, if they have low self-esteem and self-worth, chances are, their children will too. Children will mimic their parents, and often end up having similar relationships and repeating patterns with money and careers.

There is no doubt that most parents are doing the best they can with what they have, and depending on their own childhood programming, some will raise more grounded children than others. If you have children at home, then carrying out a house healing, and addressing the patterns and beliefs from your childhood, could be one of the most beneficial things you could do. For yourself, your children, and indeed, for your relationship with them.

Even if they are teenagers or older, it will still help, you could possibly prevent them from passing the same detrimental programming on to their own children that may, potentially lead to the same dysfunctional relationship.

As parents, we need to have a greater understanding of how we treat our children as we bring them into this world. We need to become far more aware of how our actions can influence them in their later life. We need to encourage them, let their minds expand. We should not impose our own fears and prejudices or indeed try and live our own lives through them.

It is said that the lessons you learn from your parents during the first five to six years of your life are like a blueprint, and they determine your thoughts and actions for the rest of your time on this planet. If fear has been the driving force at the time of your birth, then fear will play a major part in your life.

So, we need to look carefully at the legacy, that we as parents, leave our children. Also, the patterns that we may have inherited from our mothers and fathers, perhaps totally superfluous in today's modern world, that can easily leave you feeling dissatisfied, unhappy and needing therapy.

One of the things we will look at healing is our ancestral DNA, which I believe makes a huge difference in changing family patterns and programming, therefore creating a new reality for the next generations.

# Divorce & Family Separation

Just as the detrimental energies in the home can affect our programming and our health, they can also adversely affect our relationships. There were many times in my career as an Estate Agent where I came across a 'divorce house'. A home that would come up for sale every three years, like clockwork, with yet another couple separating and moving out. It was these repeating patterns of the 'divorce house' that nudged me in the direction of house healing, mainly because I wanted to find out why this was happening and what could be done about breaking this unhappy cycle.

What I found, was that you could take a happy, solid couple, put them in one of these houses, and within months their relationship would start to break down. Communication stopped, arguments became the norm, and, in some cases, paranoia set in, one or other of the couple would feel that their spouse was cheating on them. Most of these problems were caused by the noxious and inherited energies left in the house by past owners and their families.

Sometimes the energy patterns of the earth caused the initial disruption, triggering a lack of sleep, leaving the family feeling permanently tense and unsettled in their home. Over time they became irritable and short-tempered, this combined with the emotional upsets and anxiety left by past owners and their children during their divorce, created a potent cocktail of energies that always resulted in a separation.

It makes me wonder; just how many couples have divorced when it wasn't necessary? That if their home had been cleared, healed and harmonised, their relationship may well have survived? Divorce rates have rocketed in recent years, and with the additions of technopathic stress (4G and 5G etc) and the general pressure of modern life, it is really no surprise.

So, even if you have a great relationship with your spouse, it is still a good idea to carry out a healing of your home using the methods in this book. Even if it just to make sure that there are no inherited detrimental energy patterns that are affecting you, whether from past owners, visiting family, friends and, of course, any power artefacts that you have in your home.

If you have moved home recently and find that you are not sleeping well, feel more irritable than normal and tempers flare at the slightest provocation, then these could all be signs pointing to the fact that you are under the influence of detrimental energy patterns.

By removing these external influences, we can be sure that any decisions we make about our relationships are based on how we actually feel and are not being influenced by old energy patterns left behind by someone else, or due to an attachment or spirit.

# Spirituality and Business

If you have picked up this book because you feel that it is your workplace that needs healing, not your home, then these methods will work just as well for your business or office. I work with businesses as much as I do with homes. Offices, shops, warehouses, restaurants and pubs all suffer similar problems.

Stress lines, entities, attachments and many of the other issues we will be looking at, can affect concentration, productivity, attitude and in turn, the profit and health of the business. Ever wonder why some buildings keep coming up for rent and when yet another business goes under? Or why some businesses have plenty of customers, yet others struggle to entice people through the door?

It can be tricky, combining spirituality and healing with business, and there are some who believe that they should be kept separate. But I believe that a healthy, harmonious workplace is far more likely to produce the desired outcomes that the company wants, and so these issues cannot be ignored.

I gave up my commercial business to be able to totally concentrate on the healing work that I now do, but most people don't find themselves in that position, especially when they have a mortgage, children at private schools, or bank loans for the business. The pressure is always on.

I believe there is a place for mindfulness in the workplace. But trying to instil a greater understanding of other people's needs and feelings in a competitive office is not easy, especially where individual commissions are at stake, and this can create a dog-eat-dog atmosphere.

As a spiritually aware boss you do not need to discard your business suit for robes, you do not need to have statues of the Buddha in your office and you do not need to start meditating on the warehouse floor. Subtlety is the key here and this is where this book comes in.

You can work through the checklist, find the problem areas, and apply the healing methods remotely and no one would ever have to know. It is always interesting, when healing has been carried out in workplaces, without the staff being consciously aware, to observe the changes, however subtle, in their behaviour, maybe a rise in productivity or less time off for sickness.

As changes happen you will have proof that it is not simply the placebo effect at work, but that a real energetic shift has taken place.

Once you have carried out a healing, and the dynamics have shifted, some improvements may still be necessary. You could look at practical ways to help the members of staff who may be overwhelmed or struggling, by introducing some form of mentoring scheme or potentially implement a less competitive way to motivate them to improve their performance.

To get the very best from someone is what we should be striving to achieve, and it can be difficult getting an office of individuals to work together as a cohesive unit, but it can be done.

Do not forget that everyone has baggage, people bring their worries and concerns into work and these detrimental energies can be left behind when they go home, to affect others in many different ways. Their homes may well be detrimentally affected by geopathic stress and therefore they may be also bringing toxic energy patterns in with them.

I would recommend you checking the work environment periodically, carrying out a healing, clearing away any detrimental energies that may have been brought in, especially if the workplace is also open to the public. As they sit down the chairs will absorb whatever worries or concerns that they might have and, of course, as they go, they will leave some of their anxieties behind them, and these may affect your staff. In which case, I would recommend a weekly sweep.

## Case Study: Spirits with Style

I worked closely with a well-known salon owner who needed help with his staff. Several of his stylists complained about the sudden onset of splitting headaches during the day, and this led to a lot of unscheduled time off, resulting in them having to cancel clients' appointments. The salon owner was not happy.

I asked to look at his appointments book. Several of his clients booked in weekly and would see the same two stylists, who were very good and much sought after, and so a pattern was emerging. I asked if the stylists were at the top of the list for absenteeism and he said yes, he also mentioned that the trainees, responsible for hair washing and scalp massage, were also badly affected.

They were working directly within the client's auric field, allowing the worries, anxieties and stress trapped there to affect them, and they also had direct contact with client's skin, via their scalp, allowing all sorts of detrimental energies to attach themselves to the unsuspecting member of staff.

It was a simple case of carrying out a healing or clearing on the staff concerned and then talking to them about the detrimental effects of other people's emotions and how they could be transferred to each of them by working in such close proximity to their clients. I discussed various ways that they could psychically protect themselves whilst working, keeping them safe and secure during the day. It wasn't easy and, understandably, I was met with a lot of blank looks and disbelief, but a number of them agreed to do as I suggested for a week to see if it made any difference.

I went into the Salon for the first two mornings to show the staff how easy it was to bring the coloured protection into their lives. In less than ten minutes, each had completed their daily exercise and were then fully protected. I was invited to their staff meeting at the end of a busy week, to find out how they had fared. Four of the staff that protected themselves every day gave me a thumbs up. No headaches, and they also reported how much happier they felt both at the salon and at home. The other members of staff were a mixed bag, some said that they had carried out the protection for a couple of days then forgotten to do so again whilst others just hadn't bothered.

I could fully understand their reticence as I am sure that it all sounded like mumbo jumbo, but the staff who had religiously protected themselves each day had noticed a difference and had put in a full week's work with no sick days.

The salon owner was delighted that his four top stylists had taken on board what I had taught them and was very pleased with the results. So much so, that he ensured all of his staff sat as a group each morning and carried out their protection together. I monitored this for a few months, helping to fine tune the meetings. Absenteeism was then at an all-time low, the staff were so much happier, and the salon had never been busier.

Several of the staff came to see me individually as they wanted to know more about how they could help their clients. I worked with them for several months and they gradually incorporated what I had taught them into their work.

At the same time as they were cutting the clients' hair, they were giving them healing, but they were always taught to use the phrase 'as appropriate' when doing so, as this is an important point to remember, allowing Upstairs to decide on what is necessary.

Caring for your staff, in many people's eyes, can be seen as a weakness. To motivate, they use the threat of redundancy, withholding money if targets haven't been met, and constant criticism. But where is the humanity in that? I have found, over the years, that healing detrimental energies and helping staff to protect and care for themselves works far better in the long run.

You can achieve so much by treating people kindly. It's true that sometimes it might backfire on you and people may start to take advantage of your generosity and thoughtfulness. But time and time again you will be rewarded with a happier workforce who will produce more business than before you had your change of attitude.

Pay one of your small suppliers a month early, just because you can. Give your staff bonuses when they are doing well. Give someone the day off because they need to tend to personal business, without questioning them.

Spread kindness and let us see a new humility enter the business world, maybe we can get the slogan 'Do as you would be done by' displayed in every shop, office and workplace in the world.

They say that a smile can travel the globe, I believe kindness can too.

Dowsing can also be used in business in other ways too, not just to check for and heal detrimental energies, as the following case study demonstrates.

## Case Study: GHQ - The Double Agents

A practical and very drinkable use for dowsing. Although describing the serious side of dowsing, the following article is written with the advertising theme of the brand in mind.

I have worked with James (not Bond, I hasten to add) on many projects over the years, but none so much fun as when he told me that he was setting up a new company called GHQ (General Headquarters – a term used in all good spy novels during the Cold War era).

His mission: To distil and market a new and unique blend of gin and a blend of vodka from a secret and undisclosed location in Scotland.

James had spent time researching and deciphering the myriad of botanicals that were available to him, gradually decrypting them leaving a choice of twelve different runs of gin and the same number of vodkas.

Now came the difficult part, the final decision on what blends to choose.

Tasting was the obvious route to take, but due to Covid 19 and the resulting travel restrictions it was impossible for me to get to GHQ to help James. Also, for part of the journey I would have been blindfolded, because only a precious few know the location.

James carried out dozens of socially distanced blind tasting sessions with local gin and vodka lovers and friends, each scoring the individual blends finally narrowing it down to twelve.

James and his local experts had already chosen their favourite blend of gin and their favourite blend of vodka, but he asked me, via a coded message, to dowse to see what I felt would be the best of the twelve blends available. I worked through a number of questions including 'the best taste for a modern palette', 'which was going to be the most commercial', 'which left the best aftertaste', 'which was best drunk by itself', and 'which would taste better mixed with tonic'.

I rated the twelve blends of the gin and the vodka between 0 and +10, sending James the results, on paper that would self-destruct after reading.

My number one choice for each, from dowsing the twelve blends of gin and twelve of vodka, were exactly the same as those chosen not only by James but dozens of other people during their blind tasting sessions.

As James said to me afterwards 'This gives so much gravitas to your dowsing work as there were literally dozens of people here physically trying and scoring all the blends and you nailed it in one, and from a distance'.

I am very proud of the results and honoured to be part of bringing a new product to the marketplace through dowsing.

Both the gin and vodka are available for mail order via James website.

**www.ghqspirits.com**

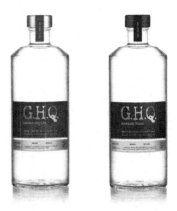

The double agents.

# Regrets

I have often heard people say, 'If I could go back to when I was 28 and change what happened, I would do so.' I guess that there are many people in the world who feel like that, but if you did go back, who would you be today and where would you be? Everybody has regrets, whether it's about the person that they should or shouldn't have married, the business opportunity that they missed, a certain friend that they should have kept in touch with but didn't, or perhaps an unsolved family rift.

Life is never perfect, or is it? All our experiences from the past make us who we are today, any slight change and you would probably be a very different person. And that doesn't necessarily mean a better person either.

We need to look at who we were and what we did, then embrace those experiences, as they enabled us to become who we are today. There are some things that can scar people for life, not just physically but mentally and spiritually too, and those events can be very difficult to deal with as there can be so many layers to peel back, many of them very uncomfortable to work through.

This is where dowsing and healing can help, clearing away many of those dark memories that have lodged themselves into our reptilian cortex, the oldest part of the brain. I liken it to the Recycle Bin of a computer, because even though the program has been deleted, unless you actually erase it completely from the bin it will still be there lurking in the background.

The ideal situation is to release these old, trapped emotions without having to remember any of the events or relive any of those buried memories. Much of the healing work contained in this book and *Heal Your Home* will help to clear these detrimental patterns. There is not one specific chapter to do this however, you will need to work through the checklist entirely.

We can only ever look forward, but we can learn from the past. And hopefully, we can use that knowledge to help change our attitude for the future.

# *Reason, Season, Lifetime*

As you start on your healing journey, you may begin to find that some people become distant, or disappear from your life, almost overnight. This can be disconcerting at first, but don't let it put you off from continuing on your path to improve your life, because, as it says in this beautiful poem that I was sent many years ago called *Reason, Season, Lifetime*, it is all happening exactly as it needs to.

We are all on a journey, people come, and people go, as do our children. We learn from them and they learn from us, we cannot and should not cling on to family, friends, lovers, or partners, putting them under obligation to stay.

## Reason, Season, Lifetime

People come into your life for a reason, a season, or a lifetime.

When someone is in your life for a **REASON**, it is usually to meet a need you have expressed or just felt. They have come to assist you through a hard time, to provide you with guidance and support, to aid you physically, emotionally or spiritually. Then, suddenly, the person disappears from your life. Your need has been met; their work is done.

Some people come into your life for a **SEASON**, because your turn has come to share or grow or give back. They bring you an experience of peace or make you laugh. They give you great joy. Believe it, it is real. But only for a season.

**LIFETIME** relationships are there to teach you lifetime lessons—things you must build upon to have a solid emotional foundation. Your job is to accept the lesson, love the person and put what you have learned to use in all your other relationships.

Think about the people in your life over the years. Whether they were there for a reason, a season or a lifetime, accept them and treasure them for however long they were meant to be part of your life.

And when they are gone, be thankful for the gifts you received from them when they were here—for a reason, a season or a lifetime

# Part Two

*Preparing to Dowse*

# Preparation is Key

Before we begin to dowse and diagnose our home, we need to make sure that we do so as safely and smoothly as possible.

You can of course, just pick up a pendulum and start asking questions, but you may find that you end up creating more problems than you started with. You can easily leave yourself wide open to psychic attack, being affected by spirits and attract detrimental attachments. Therefore, please read through the preparation sections carefully, so you are equipped to deal with whatever arises when you begin to dowse.

First of all, I would ask you to proceed with an open mind and heart. If you are familiar with *Heal Your Home*, the chances are you are already receptive to what you might find, but if this is the first time that you have read my work or tried dowsing, I encourage you to take off the blinkers and to explore the unknown without prejudice. The trick is to be sceptical and responsive at the same time.

It's easy for us to be stuck in our ways; change is not always something that we embrace with open arms, and this applies to all areas of life, not just the healing realms. I have often noticed that people involved in complementary therapies find change the most difficult, especially when it comes to their long-practiced methods and processes.

I have no doubt that our teachers, lecturers, tutors, and mentors aim to start us on our paths, pointing us in the right direction, providing us with the tools, information, knowledge, and the confidence to have a go ourselves. But energies change and we need to be aware of this fact, constantly evolving and fine tuning what we do, not necessarily rigidly following, what we have been taught in the past. There is always room for change, improvement and advancement.

There will probably be processes in this book that challenge the way you have been taught, and the healing methods that you employ in your practice, and I would ask that you remain open to trying them. Then, once you and your clients have both seen and felt the benefits, you can start to incorporate them into your daily routine, adjusting them as you see fit.

Can you remember the first time you drove a car on your own, after passing your driving test? Slightly scared, a little hesitant, your self-confidence was somewhere in the back seat? You return home from your drive, unscathed, with a big grin on your face. Well, performing a healing session by yourself for the first time can feel very much the same way.

My first distant healing session felt just like that. I had my notes open in front of me so that I didn't make a mistake, I went through each step religiously and then repeated it again, just in case I didn't get it right the first time. Did I really think that Upstairs was so pernickety that a) they didn't hear my request first time and b) I had to follow the notes exactly otherwise it wouldn't work?

Of course, this isn't the case. And after a while, I developed my own healing style and processes, and this is something I very much encourage my own students to do too.

I can understand how I felt and how others must feel when taking those first steps, but if you have good intentions and are sending unconditional love from the heart, then you will be accepted and listened to by the Universe. So, do not be afraid to release old beliefs or processes, and develop new ones.

My belief codes have changed so much over the years, as have my methods of healing. Though confidence helps and so does knowledge, you still cannot beat simply having a go. Ensure you are fully protected psychically first and then start sending loving, or healing, thoughts to someone that you know who needs help. This could simply be visualising a beam of white light filling their body with healing (entering through their crown chakra), surrounding them with a bubble of protective white light, or purely asking that they be in good health. Then wait to see what happens, it might take a while to hear but you will get feedback.

## Do we need someone's permission to send healing?

Sending love and healing leads to a question that often comes up during talks or my training courses, which is 'Do we need to ask for people's permission before we send them healing?' My answer is that in most cases you do not. Again, this may directly contradict what you have been taught in your training or mentoring, but I will explain why I believe this.

First of all, where do you think the healing comes from, you? Or Spirit?

In the past, many healers did not know about channelling energy from Spirit (the Universe/Upstairs), and they used their own internal energies to send healing to family, friends and clients. This, very quickly, led to a depletion of their own energy, they quickly became ill and many have, sadly, passed away at too early an age.

Today, we are better informed, the knowledge of how healing works is more readily available to us. We know how to tune in to Spirit, channelling the abundant, and freely available, healing (cosmic) energy through ourselves sending it, appropriately, out to others, often over vast distances, with no damage to ourselves.

I believe that Spirit has complete control over this healing. If they do not want a person to receive it then it will not happen, it doesn't matter what you do or say, it won't get through. The ultimate decision is theirs to make, you are just the conduit (middleman or woman). It doesn't matter if you have someone's full permission to send healing, if Spirit doesn't want that to happen you are powerless to do anything about it. Spirit, ultimately, sees the bigger picture, and the true pathway that the individual is treading, we do not.

I always ask that the appropriate healing is sent, and then Spirit decides how and when it will happen. If it is not the right time, whether you have that person's permission or not, the healing will not get through. I therefore only ever ask permission from Spirit before I carry out a healing, not the individual person.

I encourage you to always seek ways to improve your healing, use different techniques to see which feels best for you as one size certainly does not fit all.

When I began my journey, I was taught to connect with Spirit or the Universe, and no one at that time said anything to me about the powerful healing energy of Mother Earth, the sun or moon. After a meditation, I was informed that I must also always connect with these three heavenly beings before I carry out any form of healing. I do believe that linking to or joining with these four very powerful energies has increased my capabilities and honed my skills further.

The 21st century has changed us energetically. In the past, people had more time to dedicate themselves to healing. Holding a sweat lodge for instance, is not a five-minute event, and conducting a Druidic ceremony takes time as do most forms of Shamanistic healing.

Today we have not got the luxury of time, life is moving too fast. I do feel, that in order to fit a healing practice into our busy lives, we are allowed to streamline what we do. It is not necessarily looking for shortcuts but finding or developing quicker ways to resolve a problem. By looking at each aspect of your healing, you may find that is there an easier and quicker way to clear a blockage or remove an attachment from a client.

We are not talking about taking liberties here but trying to fine tune and speed up the healing process for the good of our clients, families, and friends. Look to see if could you use the energies that you are channelling in a different and more effective way?

It is also helpful to frequently challenge your spiritual beliefs to see if they need to be updated or improved. It is good to question them, as they may well be limiting your spiritual growth. In the early days of my 'spiritual awakening' (or perhaps 'spiritual awareness' is a better phrase to use), I said to myself 'Everything that I have read about Spirituality is complete nonsense, there are no such things as Chakras, Archangels or

Auras. Crystals don't work, God doesn't exist, etc.' I rejected all of the fundamental beliefs in the New Age society.

Then, through dowsing, I started to ask questions, and from the answers that I received began to reconstruct my beliefs, to more or less what they are today. I do still modify these as I go along, as it is a lifelong process. I believe that keeping an open mind and have a willingness to change helps to reinforce your connection with Upstairs.

I now believe in Chakras, the spinning energy centres that run throughout the body, vibrating with different colours. And there are indeed Archangels, each with their own specialities. Some are good to help with physical healing, some for mental and spiritual healing, and other for relationship problems. I am also very aware of my aura and work on keeping it clear of any nasties. I work with crystals and yes, God does exist, but not as I originally thought. I could not carry out the healing work that I do if it wasn't for my connection to the divine power.

So, if my beliefs can make a complete about turn, I believe it is possible for anyone to change. So even if you feel like yours are set in stone, pick up a pendulum and start asking questions. It doesn't hurt to be a little sceptical but do try and keep an open mind as you could be surprised by some of the answers that you receive. It will help for you to write them down in a notebook for reading later on in your development, as you may not fully understand the information that you have been given at this stage.

# Psychic Protection

If you have ever attended one of my *Heal Your Home* courses, or heard me speak, you will know that one of the main things I try to hammer home, is the need to look after yourself. Because you are the most important person in your life.

I often say, 'If all that you take away from this weekend's course is knowing the importance of Psychic Protection, and making it part of your daily practice, both for you and your family, then I have done my job'.

I cannot stress enough the importance of this daily regime. It doesn't take long, and you will feel so much better after you have worked through the process. It not only keeps you safe, but it also clears your physical body of attachments (and much more), cleanses your aura and then protects you with a multitude of colours. I also recommend going through the process with children, who are so open and sensitive. It helps them to build healthy energy protection habits.

For those of you who bought *Heal Your Home*, you will see that I have added three further colours to the meditation. Brown for your feet chakras, red ochre for your knee chakras and aquamarine for your thymus chakra (aka upper heart chakra). All are gathered into your solar plexus chakra before expanding through the physical body to the outer limits of your auric field. A kaleidoscope of spiritual colours, keeping you safe and secure.

If you keep your aura (the energetic force-field surrounding you) strong and clear, any detrimental energies that you come across will effectively bounce off. With a strong aura, it will be much harder to be 'psychically attacked' or be affected by other people's detrimental emotions.

We humans are very complex energetic beings, and when we ask a simple question while dowsing or during meditation, our energy state changes. Effectively, we open-up to explore the Universe and receive responses. Our energy centres - chakras - open to allow us to work and receive the necessary responses to our queries. This opening up can leave you susceptible to being attacked or influenced by external detrimental forces, so it is imperative that you prepare and protect yourself before you begin to diagnose and heal your home, and preferably, every day thereafter.

Whenever I mention Ouija boards to anyone, they recoil and say they would never use one for fear of attracting some evil spirit. But what they do not realise, is that dowsing opens up the same doorways. The dial that you use on a Ouija board is just the same as a dowsing rod or pendulum. You ask a question, and the rods or pendulum moves, as does the pointer. The only difference tends to be the first question.

Normally when using a Ouija board, people ask, 'Is there anybody out there?' and there normally is. If you are lucky, it will be a friendly spirit but, in many cases, it is not, and chaos ensues. When dowsing, you tend to ask specific questions, so there is less likelihood of you attracting an unfriendly or mischievous spirit, but it is still a possibility.

With Ouija boards, as with dowsing, a doorway has been opened and when the communication is finished it needs to be shut firmly. A simple *'I ask that any doorways that have been opened expectedly or unexpectedly during my dowsing/healing work are now firmly closed'*, either said out loud or in your head, should do it.

I will talk about this in more detail when we get to the healing section, but for those of you who like to dive straight in, please bear this in mind as you work through the book. As a rule, you don't go outside without a coat on when it's raining, the same rule should apply to psychic protection.

The audio version (and pdf) of the following updated Psychic Protection, is downloadable from my website www.dowsingspirits.co.uk/store.

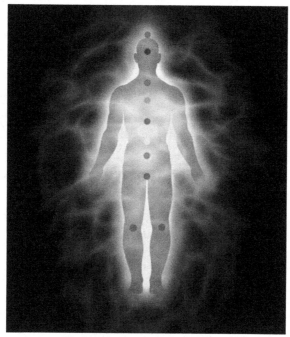

*Chakra placements on the body*

## Psychic Protection Method

We will be focusing on ten chakras for this process. Each chakra vibrates at a different frequency and each one responds to different wavelengths of light. Therefore, each has its own associated colour. They are positioned at various intervals along our 'pranic tube' which runs down through the body. It runs from the Universe above, through our crown chakra (top of the head), down the centre of our body through our base chakra and into the Earth.

For this process, we will use the solar plexus chakra as our centre point. Each colour we breathe in through each chakra will gather there, at a cellular level, and when we exhale, it expands, moving through our physical body, cleansing it of everything detrimental to us. It then continues to the outer edge of our auric field, cleansing that too. Each colour we breathe in and expand outwardly will then shrink, forming bands of protection around our body.

43

Before we start, we need to request that the following happens each time we breathe out the specified colour:

**'I ask that, as I breathe out, my body (at cellular level) and aura are cleared of all detrimental and inappropriate attachments, all lower animal life forms, their seeds and tentacles, all human manifested thought forms and life forms, all worries and concerns, any miasms and detrimental family DNA, any cancers and tumours, any past, present and parallel life traumas or upsets, all detrimental parental patterning, all parasites and any other detrimental energies that are inappropriate to me. I also request that all unnecessary psychic and physical cords are cut and that everything that has been removed or dislodged is taken into the light and disposed of appropriately. I ask that the healing takes place not only in this dimension but all other dimensions that are similarly affected.'**

Once you have made the above request, either silently or out loud, sit quietly and take two deep breaths.

First, visualise breathing in the colour **brown** through the chakras on the soles of your feet. See this moving up your legs to your solar plexus, via your pranic tube, then forming a glowing ball of light at cellular level. As you breathe out, visualise it expanding through your body to the outer edge of your auric field, cleansing the body and aura of all detrimental and inappropriate energy patterns. It then shrinks to form a two-inch layer of brown around your physical body, this is your connection to Mother Earth.

Then breathe in **red ochre (reddish brown)** through the chakras found in each knee. Bring this up to your solar plexus through both legs, and your body via your pranic tube. From here, see it expanding through your body to the outer edge of your aura, cleansing both of all detrimental energy patterns. It then shrinks to form a two-inch layer of reddish brown around your physical body, outside the brown protective barrier.

Next breathe in **red**, through your base chakra and up into your solar plexus via your pranic tube. At the top of your breath, exhale. Expand this healing colour through your body to the edge of your aura, cleansing both of all detrimental energy patterns and then it shrinks to form a third layer around you, over the red ochre barrier.

Next breathe in **orange**, through your sacral chakra and up into your solar plexus via your pranic tube. At the top of your breath, exhale. Expand this healing colour through your body to the edge of your aura, cleansing both of all detrimental energy patterns and then it shrinks to form a fourth layer around you, over the red.

Next breathe in **yellow**, through your solar plexus chakra. At the top of your breath, exhale, pushing the healing light through your body to the outer edge of your aura. This cleans all detrimental energy patterns, shrinking to form a fifth layer around you, over the orange barrier, just like the layers of an onion.

Breathe **green** in through your heart chakra, and down into your solar plexus via your pranic tube. As you exhale, push the colour through your body to the outer edge of your auric field, cleansing the body and aura. It then shrinks, to form a sixth layer around you.

Breathe **aquamarine** into your thymus (or upper heart) chakra and feel it moving down to your solar plexus. Exhale and push the colour through your body to the outer edge of your auric field – cleansing it. Then allow it to shrink to form the seventh layer around you.

Breathe in **light blue** through your throat chakra down into your solar plexus via your pranic tube. Exhale to push the colour through your body and aura, then shrink it to form the eighth layer.

Breathe **dark blue** in through your third eye/brow chakra down into your solar plexus via your pranic tube. Exhale to push the colour through your body and aura, then shrink to form a ninth layer.

Through your crown chakra, breathe in **purple** sending it down to your solar plexus. Exhale to cleanse the body and aura, then see it shrink to become the tenth protective layer.

Then breathe in a **silver** light through your crown chakra, into your solar plexus. Exhale, and push it through your body and aura. It shrinks to form the eleventh layer.

Breathe in a **gold** light, via your crown chakra, into your solar plexus and as you exhale push it through your body and aura, cleansing them of all detrimental energy patterns. It shrinks to form the twelfth and final protective barrier.

45

Finally breathe in **divine white light**, via your crown chakra, see it filling up your body from the tips of your toes to the top of your head. You can, if you wish, push it out to fill the whole of your aura.

You are now fully protected; your chakras are cleansed, as is your body and auric field.

If you ever find yourself unable to sleep, try this exercise. You may find that you never reach your crown chakra, and slip into a deep, energetically protected sleep.

# Spirit Guides

In *Heal Your Home*, spirit guides were mentioned in general, but the more I do this work, the more I have realised that it is important for you not just to acknowledge their presence and ask for their help, but to actually get to know who they are.

This can include finding out their names, their culture, and their history. I believe this will help you in your healing work, as I know that it has helped me with mine. There is also more information on spirit guides in my second book, *Spirit & Earth*, co-authored with Tim Walter, from which I will be borrowing small segments for this chapter. There is also new information of why and when spirit guides change and how to detect these changes.

## Who or what are our Spirit Guides?

A spirit guide is the energy of someone that you have chosen to work with or who has volunteered to be your guide during your time here on Earth. They have elected to stay in the higher realms to assist and protect you, rather than incarnating here on Earth. They will know you first as a spiritual being but also in your mortal guise. It appears that, before we incarnate, much goes on between us and those who end up being our spirit guides.

We all have spirit guides. Some will be with you from birth and stay with you throughout your incarnation on Earth. Other guides will come in at different points during your life, but there will always be a special one who will be with you for the duration. Some people consider this one to be their guardian angel.

Many of us first become aware of our spirit guides as children, because our heads are less cluttered by day-to-day concerns and we have a less blinkered view of the world. We are open to new experiences and our guides find it much easier to connect with us at this stage of our lives. As we grow older, our energies become denser as we deal with day-to-day problems, stress, relationship issues, and money worries.

It would seem that some so-called "imaginary friends" are perhaps not so imaginary. They may well in fact be spirit guides. Just because a parent cannot see them does not mean they do not exist. They will be vibrating at a different level to us, a lighter energy that the older generation are unable to connect with or visualise. I was very lucky with my parents. Ma, in particular, was very sensitive and acknowledged my 'invisible' friend called Bankinks, he came everywhere with me, he was my constant companion.

Sadly, when parents insist that there is no one there, that these imaginary friends really do not exist, it can be the start of the barriers going up between us and the higher realms, gradually cutting off our natural connection to these helpful guardian souls.

Gradually over the years, Bankinks faded away, and this, I believe, was due to the modern education system. All teachings are carried out in a very left brain (logical) way, and are about learning how to pass exams, leaving little room for intuition and sensitivity. This meant that the right-hand side of my brain (intuition and spirituality) had to take a back seat for many of my early years.

I re-established contact in my late 30s, when a spirit medium told me that my 'imaginary friend' was in fact my spiritual brother and that we'd had many lives together. This time, the medium continued, Bankinks had chosen to remain in the higher realms to help me with my spiritual development, formulate my healing techniques and strengthen my connection to the divine. I remember feeling very humbled by this information as it was given to me. I imagined Bankinks holding his hands up in the air saying, 'At last I've got him back, it's only taken 20 years!' He is with me today whilst I write this book, as are my other guides.

You will find that different guides will come and go, depending on what stage you have reached in your spiritual development. They will help you move forward, and as you advance, reaching the next stage, they can leave, to be replaced by one or more new guides, normally more powerful than the last.

But some, like Bankinks, will remain for the duration.

## Connecting to your Spirit Guide

Initially, meditation is the key to making a conscious connection to your guides. But do not expect a 'wow' moment the first time you do this, because it can take time. Also, please do not be put off if the results aren't what you expect or hope for, and make sure that you have carried out the psychic protection exercise before you do the following meditation, or any meditation for that matter. Have a pen and paper ready to make notes after you finish.

## The Spirit Guide Meditation

Sit with both feet flat on the floor, get comfortable, switch off your mobile phone and make sure that you will not be disturbed for at least thirty minutes. If you wish music playing in the background that is perfectly okay as it can help drown out any unwanted noises.

I would always suggest, that before you carry out any form of meditation, that you psychically protect yourself, it guarantees your wellbeing, and it is always better to be safe than sorry.

Begin to quieten the mind and body, take a few deep breaths, counting your breaths as you inhale and exhale, and start to relax. Continue counting your breaths for as long as you need in order to quieten your mind. Gradually you will feel the calmness spreading from within. As you do so, picture yourself walking along a path, it does not matter where it is, the choice is yours.

Feel the air around you, become aware of the sounds around you, perhaps the birds are singing, bees buzzing or there is a gentle murmur of faraway traffic. Feel the ground underneath your feet. How does it feel? Rough or smooth? Is it a pavement, gravel, or soil? Concentrate on walking along it. Feel the sunshine on your back, the natural warmth of the day.

A short way off, you see a woodland and the path that you are on takes you into it. As you walk amongst the trees, the leaves cast dappled shadows on the ground. These shadows become more pronounced the deeper into the woodland you go, until there is nothing but darkness. Do not worry as you are fully protected.

In the distance, you see a tiny pinprick of light. You walk towards it, gradually becoming aware that the sun is once again shining through the leaves and then suddenly you emerge from the dark of the woodland into a lush green meadow.

You stop and take your shoes and socks off. Instantly, you feel the connection to Mother Earth. You feel grounded. You become aware of the healing energy moving up your legs, passing through your feet, knees, base and sacral chakras and into your solar plexus chakra where it is held as a glowing ball of light.

Then you become aware of a magnificent light shining from above, entering your crown chakra, passing through your third eye (brow), throat, thymus, and heart chakras, entering your solar plexus chakra where it mixes with the healing light from Mother Earth.

The Sun's energy then enters from the front and back of your solar plexus chakra meeting and mixing with the other healing energies stored there. Finally, the moon sends down her heavenly light which envelops your whole body and then condenses into the solar plexus where all the energies merge together.

The glowing ball of light starts to expand, through your cells, bloodstream, major organs, skin, chakras and so on until it has completely cleared your body of all detrimental energies. It continues to move through your aura until it has reached its extremity.

Once it is there, ask that all the detrimental energies that have been dislodged be taken into the light and disposed of in the most appropriate way.

Now that you are clear of all detrimental energies you are ready to meet your spirit guide. You look around and see an open-air temple close by, and you walk towards it. You descend a few stone steps and find yourself in front of an altar bedecked with flowers and lit candles, you are bathed in the light. There, a few steps away, there is a wooden bench with two cushions placed on it. You walk to it and sit. You slowly become aware of how peaceful you feel, how much a part of the whole you have become.

You start to become conscious of an energetic presence near you. As you focus your attention and awareness you see your spirit guide beginning to appear, first as an ethereal shimmer and then taking solid form.

You are now in the presence of an amazing being. You might recognise them from childhood. They sit beside you and take hold of your hand. You feel the connection as the energy moves through your body. As this happens you may hear them giving you a message or possibly a gift to bring back with you.

Stay for as long as you wish, the energies here will be very beneficial to you.

Once you decide to leave your spirit guide, stand up, turn to them, put your hands together, over your heart as in prayer, bow and thank them for being with you today and give gratitude for the help and support they have given you over the years.

Leave the temple and walk back along the meadow, stopping to put your shoes and socks on. At the edge of the meadow, just before the woodland, on your right-hand side, you will see a 'spiritual wheelie bin'. Open it and dispose of any old thoughts, worries and stresses that you no longer need or want to bring back home with you.

Re-enter the woodland, noticing once again the dappled shadows on the pathway. Keep walking, once again it gets darker and darker until you reach almost pitch black. Then, in the distance, you see that pinprick of light and you keep moving towards it. Your surroundings become lighter and lighter until you find yourself back in the sunshine and on your original pathway.

Follow this until you are back in your room. Take some time to 'come to', take a few breaths and then when you are ready, open your eyes.

In this first meeting with your spirit guide you might not see, hear or feel anything but don't give up. Repeat this process as soon and as often as you can. The more you do it, the easier it will become for both you and your spirit guide to make meaningful contact.

Write down your experience, remembering any little thing you can about your travels and the visit to see your spirit guide. Make a note of their appearance, what they might have said and what gift they may have given you. Add to this each time you meditate. By doing so you will be able to see how your connection is changing and improving each time you meet.

I would suggest that you check on your guides every few months to see if there has been a change. The more healing work that you do, the more chance you will have of a new guide coming through. If you have bought my book to purely work on your own home, then checking on your guides regularly may not be a necessity for you.

I would always suggest connecting with your main guides first as they can protect you. They are the most important ones and finding out who they are keeps you safe. Once you are happy that you have connected with your main guides, you can then start to tune into your protection guides.

## How do we know when our spirit guides have changed?

It can sometimes be a feeling; you may hear a clearly spoken message or receive several subliminal images or sounds. Or you may not notice the shift at all.

My guides had been with me for several years when I became aware of changes in energies as I connected with them, during my daily ritual before I started my healing sessions.

### First Change:

Several years ago, I was mentoring Tim and we were working on a house in the USA. During our work we picked up on three spirits that needed moving into the light, one of whom was a Native American Chief/

Shaman. He told us that he was the Guardian of the Land and had been for many generations, but it was his time to go. He refused to be moved on along with the other two spirits though, as in his own eyes, he was too important and wanted an individual ceremony. So that is what we did. He moved on and I thought that would be the last we would see of him.

That was until about two years later when I suddenly got the urge to read books and watch television programmes featuring Native Americans and their culture. Often, when I am conducting a healing session, I have Buddhist monks chanting in the background, but that suddenly did not seem appropriate anymore. During my meditations I was hearing different drums beating, the chanting was no longer from Nepal or Tibet, it was Native American.

So, I started dowsing and asked if what I was hearing was significant and got a yes.

*Is it to do with my guides? Yes.*

*Have I got a new guide coming in? Yes.*

*Is one leaving me? Yes.*

I dowsed and found that the Benedictine Monk, who had been with me for several years, had gone on to pastures new to make way for this new person.

Have I come across this guide before in my healing work? Yes.

*Is it a male or female? Male.*

*What continent is he from? USA.*

*Have I helped him go to the light in the past? Yes.*

Then it clicked. The Native American books, the TV programmes, the drums.

*Is it the important Shaman that Tim and I moved through some years back? Yes.*

*Wow* was my very first thought. I needed to find out his name. I tuned in and asked him to come close and tell me what I should call him.

His name? Eagle That Soars.

## Second Change:

The second change took place not long after the first, but rather than hearing different music, I was guided by smell.

I tend to burn a lot of sage incense in my healing room as I work, but one day it just did not feel right to do so. The room felt stuffy and claustrophobic, my nose was blocked, and my head felt like it was stuffed with cotton wool. Initially I put it down to hay fever.

I went out into the garden, I grounded and cleared myself then my healing room, just in case anything had slipped through the daily protection that I always surround the house with. I went back inside and still felt the same way. I asked Upstairs whether something was wrong, and they said no, everything was okay, spiritually.

So, I meditated and asked the following questions:

*Is it hay fever? No.*

*Was it the incense that caused the problem? Yes*

*Was the problem with the incense significant? Yes.*

*Physically or spiritually? Spiritually.*

*If I changed the incense, would that help? Yes.*

*Which incense do I need to burn? I was given a mental picture of an incense that I had bought on one of my visits to India.*

I had to stop the meditation and search for the packet of incense sticks, and as I lit the taper the energies suddenly changed, felt much lighter and brighter, and the heaviness disappeared.

I admit to scratching my head at this point. Sometimes you need Upstairs to throw you a lifeline, so I asked them, and they replied.

A short one-word message: Guide.

The penny dropped and I started to ask questions again:

*Do I have a new guide coming in? Yes.*

*Male of Female? Female.*

*From India? Yes.*

I asked for a clue and was given PAYE.

I wondered whether she had been an accountant or worked for the HM Revenue and Customs as it meant nothing else to me. But no, she hadn't done either job.

I looked up 'Paye' on the internet, and after scrolling down one or two pages I found the following:

Paye is a small village, located in Bhiwandi Tehsil region of the Thane district in Maharashtra, India. It is well known for the temples venerating the Goddess Sateri, but I had never heard of the village or her before.

*Is my new guide the Goddess Sateri? Yes.*

It was a double wow moment. Working with two new guides, to me, is something very special and humbling. It has certainly helped in my healing work and they have brought with them new questions to ask when carrying out house and family healings.

If you wish to find out what guides are working with you, there is a downloadable chart on my website that should assist you in dowsing for their name, background and history. It will take time and patience, but I believe it is very much worth it. You could also meditate, inviting them to visit you, asking them who they are and why they are with you.

## What Are Protection Guides?

They are a similar being to a spirit guide as they are spirit, but their job is very different. They protect you in day-to-day life as well as when you carry out any form of healing, whereas the other guides are more like teachers, guiding and helping you with your spiritual development.

I am fully aware of their existence and call on them every day to be with me, especially when carrying out any healing, but strangely I had never thought to find out anything further about them until I started writing this book.

I have now delved deeper, meditated, and found out who they are and what their job description is. I believe that this knowledge will help deepen the quality of my healing work even further.

I was born with massive protection around me, but I did not know this until I was lucky enough to meet John Benedict, a world-renowned palmist. I had gone to him seeking advice about my estate agency business that was having difficulties during the recession in the late 1980s. He took one look at my hands and said that he had never seen such large protection triangles on anyone before, that I was being very well looked after and was destined to become a healer.

I certainly did not expect to hear anything like that. I felt both honoured and confused, however, looking back I realise that John had lit the blue touch paper, and after that it was simply a waiting game until Upstairs called me. He did say that the protection given to me would last until my early 40s, and after that time I would have to start taking control of my own spiritual health. I admit to doing a lot of reading after hearing that, to find out how to do so effectively.

What John did not tell me until much later is that I had a strong protection guide with me all the time and still do, but he wanted me to delve into the spiritual realms and this was his way of encouraging me to do so.

All but one of my protection guides have been replaced as my healing work has progressed and become more intricate. I now have three protection guides, all of whom are all women.

One has been with me since I started my healing work, she is my strongest supporter, refers to herself as my Gatekeeper and it is she that keeps me safe, sending me the work that she knows I can deal with.

Now, her trust in me was greater than the belief I had in myself, especially in the very early days. Some of the things I have had to deal with over the years have been terrifying and certainly not something that I would have actively sought to have taken on myself. But I trust that she knows best. Her name is Babh and she was alive in the 8th century. She passed away in 773 AD aged 97. She was a mystic, known to have second sight and was sought after by many people at that time. That was her last incarnation on Earth, since then she has been helping people as a spirit.

She is now here for me, and apparently, for me only. She helps me with my healing work by protecting me, she is a hard task master, keeping me on my toes and sending me a lot of work. I do have to ask her to calm it down sometimes as I can get overwhelmed and tired.

I can call on her at any time that I feel unsure or have a problem that has me scratching my head as to how to deal with it. Sometimes she helps but sometimes I am left to my own devices and have to work the problem out using the knowledge that I have gained throughout my lifetime.

My second protection guide comes from Kenya and was a member of the Meru tribe. She was known as a witch but in essence she was a healer, using natural herbs to help her village. She passed away in 1341 AD aged 66 years old.

My third protector lived in what is now known as Lebanon. She was widely sought after as a soothsayer and she died in 1667 at 32 years old. She has not said how she passed, but it was not of natural causes.

So, my life is in the hands of three very powerful women, four if you include my wife, Allyson.

## How to invoke your Protection Guides

To invoke these special protection guides, proceed with belief, respect, and confidence.

Sitting still and emptying your mind is a good way to start, in other words, meditation. Ideally, before we start any form of healing, it is good to communicate with your protection guides. You may not know who they are yet but introduce yourself, either out loud on in your head, they will be listening. This helps us to bond with them, and as you start on your healing journey you will normally have one or more assigned to you. This happens naturally, without needing to request it, but it is respectful to find out more about them.

Belief that you are protected by your guides will help, but I always like to complete the protection method every day, as that shows respect and that you are able and willing to help yourself, rather than just relying purely on others to do the job for you. Upstairs loves it when people take responsibility for their own spiritual hygiene, it shows spiritual growth and understanding.

The more you connect with them, the more confidence you will gain and the easier it will become for both you and them. After a while, you will be able to invoke their help with a simple thought.

I like to sit quietly in nature. Anywhere with grass, trees or plants will do, it can be your back garden if that's all that's available. But if you have a park, woodland or river nearby then head there, so long as it is quiet. If you can find a tree to sit beside or lean your back against, even better. The connection with Mother Earth will keep you grounded but also allow you to be still and leave your thoughts behind.

## Meditation

Perform the protection method to clear your aura and then concentrate on your breath, cool as it enters your body and warm as you exhale. In and out, in and out, until you start to relax and as you do you may find your breathing is shallower than before. Just keep working with this feeling. The body and mind are as one, calm and peaceful.

Try bonding with the tree, (asking its permission first) as it is the conduit between Heaven and Earth, its roots deep in ground and its branches in the air. It is a good way to become even more serene and connected.

Set your intention to connect with your protection guide, and then allow your imagination to wander. Start by visualising the planet. You are flying above the clouds and seeing all the countries below you, is there one that draws you in? Is there a particular town or city that catches your attention, or a picture in your third or mind's eye of where your protection guide might come from? Make a mental note of where it is.

This will indicate their nationality, but if you wish to go further, ask if there is a particular building linked to your guide. Again, see if you can get a picture in your third eye, if not, do not worry, it may happen in time.

Try asking your protection guide to come forward, to meet you and be aware of any slight energetic changes that might be taking place. If you don't get flashing lights, a clash of symbols or see a complete figure standing in front of you, do not worry, again these things can take time and patience.

As with most things, and meditation is no exception, the more you practice the better you get at it. You may find colours starting to change, or you can hear a voice in your head, or see the glimpse of a face as your guide comes through. Whatever happens, or doesn't happen, send your thanks. Do not worry if nothing occurred, you have shown your willingness and intention to connect, it will get easier and better the more you try.

They will also be helping you, sending you signs that they are there. Look out for the repetition of a word or colour, or a certain song that is special to you. You can also ask for signs that you can recognise.

Now the bond is forming, you can start to ask for extra protection, whether for when you are going to work, performing a healing session, dowsing or for when you socialise. They will be with you anyway, but with your permission, they can do more to help you.

As with any meditation, take your time to come out of it and when you do ask that any doorways that were opened expectedly or unexpectedly during your meditation are firmly closed.

# Healing Energy

## How do we channel healing energy?

Once you have fully protected yourself, the next thing to ensure, before you begin the healing part of the process, is that you are not using your own energy to conduct the healing. If you do, you are asking for trouble. Maybe not in the short term but certainly in the medium to long term. If you use your own energy for healing work, your internal batteries are quickly going to be depleted and you will start to suffer from many different aches and pains lack of energy, brain fog etc. This eventually leads to a spiritual burn out.

Many healers have suffered early deaths, due to their life force having been drained away. They had freely given healing to others, but this was using their core 'inner' energy. Once it ran out there was no replenishing it.

Therefore, we need to find an external source or sources that have a limitless supply of energy that we can link into (channel), to help ourselves and to send to others. Welcome to Upstairs, the Management, The Powers that Be, the Highest of the High, God, the Universe, Jehovah, Allah or simply The Light. Feel free to call this higher power whatever you feel comfortable with or what your belief codes dictate.

To **CHANNEL** this boundless source of healing light, you simply have to call upon the higher power to send it to you, allowing it to safely enter your body, directing to whomever you are working on. Whether they are sitting right in front of you or living a thousand miles away, the effect will still be the same.

After fully protecting yourself visualise the light from the Universe (Upstairs) entering your crown chakra and flowing through your heart chakra, down your arms and out through your fingertips to the person or place you are wanting to send healing to. Or you can simply trust that the healing energy is flowing through you to where you intend it to go, if you find visualisation difficult.

## How does distant healing work?

Previously, I have travelled to work on clients' homes around the world, which is not only time consuming, but also very expensive. Therefore, for the last few years, most of my work has been carried out at a distance, from the safety of my home in the Yorkshire Dales.

In the healing section of this book you will see, and often repeated, the words 'flooding the energy line (or other problem) with light and love'. But how can someone living in the UK be able to send effective healing to a family living in, say, Australia?

Let's start with looking at what light actually is.

Light radiates from its source in waves, each wave has two parts: one electric and the other magnetic. That is why it is referred to as Electromagnetic Radiation. Interestingly, the light with shortest wavelength (purple/violet) carries far more energy than a light with long wavelengths (red).

This correlates to the chakra points of the physical body. The purple crown chakra has the highest vibration allowing the healing (light), from the 'source', to enter the body whilst the base chakra (red) is viewed as a lower vibrating energy centre.

Light travels at just over 186,000 miles a second, and in that time, it can travel seven times around the equator.

So how does that explain how healing works?

Healing energy is made of light waves and they can penetrate any object or person. So, if you imagine light coming from the Universe, being channelled through you, leaving your body and by thought being sent to the person or place you are healing, it will be there in micro-seconds, literally at the speed of light. The effects can be instantaneous, just as though the person is sitting in the same room as you.

We are literally channelling the energies of the Universe.

Scientists have been measuring the light (higher wavelengths) naturally produced by, not just our Universe, but from distant Universes. I feel that this is a major part of what healers are able to utilise, or channel, when carrying out their work.

I always keep a record of the time and date that I start my distant healing work, and I often receive emails from clients telling me exactly when the healing started. More often than not it matches, to the minute, when I began my work. But sometimes the healing is received before I start looking at the house plan and this phenomenon is looked at in greater detail later in the book.

# Dowsing

If you have ever seen someone walking across a ploughed field or farmyard with two bits of bent wire in their hands, your first thought is likely to be 'nutter'! What most people do not realise is that through those two bits of old coat hanger you are connecting to the Universe or Spirit.

People have been trying to prove, or disprove, dowsing for years and many have tried to figure out exactly how and why it works. Science likes repeatability in experiments, and that is where the case for dowsing tends to fall down. There have been tests devised over the years and in many of the cases, the dowsers taking part, have failed to provide satisfactory proof that it works.

To dowse properly you need to be in a relaxed state of mind, otherwise the answers are likely to be incorrect or inconsistent and this is what, I feel, causes the problems when under experimental conditions. How can you remain calm when you are under pressure, especially if you are desperate to prove that dowsing actually works? Failure is the most likely outcome or at best, limited success.

I have received proof, over and over, that dowsing does actually work, but rather than take my word for it, I encourage you to have a go, start to practice and test it for yourself.

Dowsing, to me, is a grounded way of connecting to Upstairs or the Universe and I believe that everyone can do it, to a greater or lesser degree. Of course, there are people who have special gifts, some are clairaudient, some clairsentient and others clairvoyant, they may find that dowsing helps develop their sensitivity and in time, may not need the rods or pendulum in order to receive answers.

When it comes to dowsing, take your time, work in a systematic and methodical way, keep yourself hydrated and stay in a calm mental state. You will probably find yourself starting to tire easily when you first pick up the rods or pendulum, this is because you are receiving a lot of information in ways that you are not used to, psychically.

But do keep at it, gradually lengthening the amount of time that you spend dowsing. You will find that the rods will become more responsive, as does the motion of the pendulum. As time goes by you may suddenly become aware that you know the answer to the question that you have just asked, even though the rods have not yet moved.

It is imperative, when dowsing a house, that you do so for all the family members, not just for you. You need to focus your mind and phrase all the questions so that each individual receives the correct healing energies. Because what affects one member of the household, may not affect everyone.

## What to look for and how to find it

Much of the diagnostic work in this book is carried out by dowsing using the question strings provided.

For more in-depth information on how to dowse, please check out *Heal Your Home* and *Spirit & Earth* as they contain detailed descriptions on how to hold and use dowsing rods and pendulums.

But as a brief reminder, if you are using rods or a pendulum, you will need to have established your 'yes' or 'no' response to get the answers to the questions in the string.

There are, of course, other forms of dowsing that you could use. For instance, I now use my eyes. They flick up for a yes response and down for no. This has taken many years to develop but is so much easier than carrying a pendulum or rods with me all the time.

You can body dowse, using a backward and forward swaying movement as your yes and no response, or a movement to one side or the other. I have even seen people use a mobile telephone swinging at the end of a lanyard as a pendulum. Any heavy object tied on to a piece of string can be used as a pendulum, but for the purpose of dowsing the questions in this book, I would suggest you have a dedicated pendulum one that you have programmed to work with you.

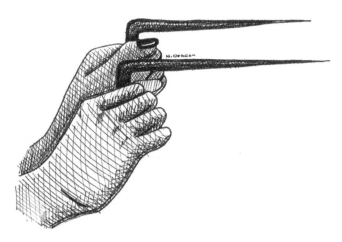

*How to hold your rods in the search position*

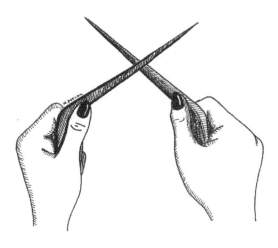

*A crossing of the rods is the general yes response from your rods; however, each person is different, and you will need to ascertain this for yourself. Do take your time.*

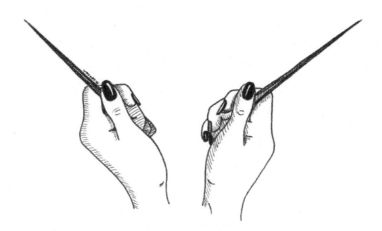

*An average no response, the rods moving in opposite directions*

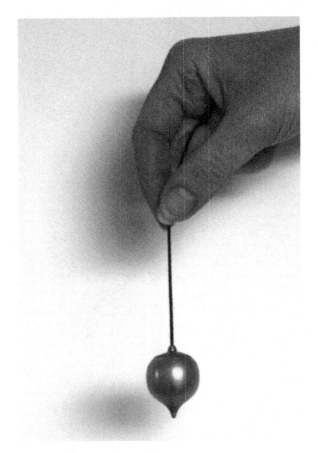

*How to hold a pendulum*

Before you start to diagnose, and if you are new to dowsing, practice makes perfect so do be patient and take your time. Start by asking a lot of verifiable questions such as:

*'Am I wearing a blue shirt today?'* Yes/No

*'Am I holding an agate pendulum (or whatever the crystal may be)?'* Yes/No

*'Is my front door painted blue/red/green?'* Yes/No

Check that you get a different response to your yes and no answers, there is no right or wrong way for the rods or pendulum to move, everyone is different. Rarely will your responses change, but an illness, a trauma in your life or a change of spirit guide can alter the direction of your yeses and no's. So, it is worth checking your responses again, by asking the questions above, or by asking for a yes or no response, before commencing a diagnostic or healing session.

To see how detrimental something is, I use a scale of 0 to -10. To get this figure I just state the numbers out loud until I get a positive reaction from the rods or pendulum but do count slowly until you are practiced enough to get an immediate reaction from your rod or pendulum. If you count too quickly you may find that you have passed the actual number before the rod or pendulum has had a chance to move. You may find it easier to begin with using the diagram below.

You start your pendulum swinging over the chart, and either out loud or in your mind, ask that it shows how detrimental, for example, one of the water veins is that you have found for you and the family. Give it a chance to settle and then see what number it is swinging over and note it down.

Exactly the same applies when using a dowsing rod, hold it over the chart, pointing straight ahead of you and ask it to show you how detrimental the water vein is to you and the family. See what number it points and note it down.

I am not one for asking, can I, may I, or should I, when it comes to dowsing, I pick up the rods or pendulum ask a question, and if I get a response then away I go. I always psychically protect myself and ask to be linked to The Highest of the High, Mother Earth, Our Life-Giving Sun and Heavenly Moon.

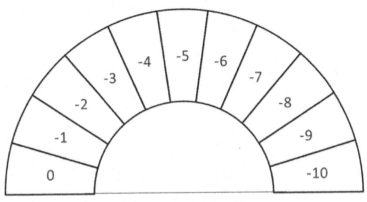

Detrimental Energy Chart

**NB** There is a free information sheet available to download on How to Dowse via the Online Shop of my website: www.dowsingspirits.co.uk.

## Dowsing and concentration

People often ask me why I seem to prefer staying at home to dowse, rather than visit a client on site.

Apart from the time and expense of travelling, first and foremost it is about safety. By working from a distance, you are not likely to be affected by the detrimental energy patterns found in someone's home. Psychic protection works, but why continually put yourself in harm's way when distant healing is often more effective than being on site.

Of course, if you are reading this with the intention of healing your own home, then you will likely be in the house whilst you are carrying out the diagnosis and healing. In which case it is imperative that you are fully protected, you can also ask the angels to help keep the detrimental energies from affecting you whilst you carry out the work.

If you begin to feel unwell at any point, stop, go outside for some fresh air, make sure you are hydrated, and then, if you feel well enough, resume. Walking in the garden barefoot can help to ground you.

Second of all, it is a question of concentration. People find dowsing fascinating and therefore, if visiting a client's house, it can be very difficult to fully focus on finding an underground pipe or a water course when they are chatting away in the background.

Understandably, people have a fascination with dowsing, especially when I am in their home or garden, and they cannot help but ask questions often want to have a go themselves. Though understandable, it can be very distracting, and it does not help my concentration or my ability to find the object that I have been asked to locate.

## Case Study: Missing Stopcock in Surrey

When I was living in Godalming, I received a telephone call from a gentleman from Guildford one morning.

'I've lost my stopcock, he said.

'Do you think it has gone far?' I said jokingly.

'No, it's in my garden and I don't know exactly where it is, could you come and locate it for me. That's what dowsers do isn't it?' he replied.

It was a nice day so I said I could come over as I was sure that it could be located quite easily. I arrived and was ushered into the kitchen and offered a cup of tea. The gentleman explained that they had refitted the kitchen recently and had a minor leak from one of the new connections. It hadn't been a major problem and could have been a lot worse. If the leak had been a bigger it would have necessitated them turning the water off at the mains, hence the reason for calling me over to locate the missing stopcock.

He told me 'The couple we bought the house from, several years back, built a rockery in the front garden, over the stopcock and although they told us where it was, we have forgotten, we have never needed to find it'.

Then he quickly switched tack and asked, 'How does this dowsing thing work then?'

The missing stopcock was forgotten about as I explained that all objects vibrate at different levels and how by tuning in (concentrating) you can find what you are looking for.

'Can I have a go?' he asked.

I passed the rods over and instructed him on how to find his yes and no responses, his wife also wanted to try them out. I had another cup of tea and talked more on dowsing related topics. Can you see where this is going?

'Okay, let's go outside now and find the missing stopcock,' I said.

We all went out to the front garden and the talking continued, 'So where do you think it is then?' he asked as he followed me around.

I asked the rods to show me where the stopcock was, they swung and pointed to the rockery, so far so good. I walked along until they crossed and pointed to a spot on the ground where the stopcock was located. Told him that is was about 24" down and marked the locating with a pebble. I had a final cup of tea and drove home.

I received a telephone call about two week later saying that due to the inclement weather he had only just got into the garden and had dug down about 3ft and found nothing. 'Shall I keep going?' he said.

'No, I think that you had better stop, I will come over tomorrow morning and see what is going on,' I replied.

My first thought was 'You've lost it, you can't dowse.' Not at all helpful, but I then started to think, how come I got it so wrong? Lack of concentration was the first thing that came into my mind. I had been unable to fully concentrate on the task at hand, as the couple had been so interested in dowsing and I had been more than willing to impart the information. Because of this, I had forgotten to clear my head and tune in. I should have politely asked them to leave me to work quietly on my own.

So, I decided to locate the house using Google Earth. I printed off the plan, then map dowsed. I quickly located the cold-water pipe coming out of the house and traced to where it joined up with the mains supply in the street. Armed with that information I travelled back to Guildford to find the missing stopcock.

I apologised for having him dig in the wrong place and politely asked him to leave me alone for five minutes as I needed that time to concentrate. I dowsed and found where the cold-water pipe came out of the house, marking that with a flag, I then followed the route of the pipe, marking every two feet with a coloured flag. The pipe ran along the front of the house before angling away, heading towards the road. I got to the rockery and the rods crossed, about 18" from where he had been digging, the exact place that I had already marked on the plan.

I called the gentleman out and told him that I had found the stopcock. I took a flag and pushed the flag into the ground, it went in about 5" and then hit metal. 'I thought you said it was 24" down?' he said. We dug away the soil and uncovered the metal cap, levered it up, and there 19" down, was the stopcock. I had found it. He was overjoyed as indeed was I.

The lesson had been learned. Concentration is so important when dowsing, you need to remain focussed and often the best way to do so is at home, in peace and quiet. It also helps to do the investigative work before you go on location, as it will pay dividends in the long run.

# Part Three

*Diagnosing Your Home*

# The New Checklist

It is important that when working on your home you do so diligently and take your time. We will be working through my complete checklist and diagnosing the detrimental energies that are affecting you, your family and home. This is the same checklist that I use daily, when working on clients' homes.

If you have read and used *Heal Your Home*, then you may notice that the questions are in a slightly different order than before. This is due to the new questions that have been included. The questions have now been all been correlated and placed into sections which, to me, is now more logical. In part four, you will see that the healing is performed in this same new order.

In the new checklist, you will find everything from the *Heal Your Home* checklist (with a few updates/amendments) along with further insights, questions and case studies. Some of the original headings have also been slightly changed, these will be explained as we work through each section.

As explained above, I have split the checklist into further sub-categories, to make it easier to understand what energies you are working with. When you start to work through the checklist, you can, if you wish, tackle just one or two categories at a time, so that you do not get overwhelmed. But I would still recommend that all the healing is performed in one go, if possible, for the best outcome.

A question that I like to ask before I start dowsing is, 'Am I going to find anything interesting or unusual?' If the answer is yes, make a note and then ask again at the end if you have found it. If not, then it could be a new topic for you to explore.

Before you begin to dowse, remember to use the Psychic Protection Method to keep yourself safe. Then at the end of each dowsing session (if you do it in parts over time) and also at the end of the healing give thanks to all the beings that have been with you and then to ensure that all doorways that have been opened are closed by saying the following statement *'I ask that all doors that were expectedly or unexpectedly opened during the healing process are now firmly closed'*.

As you begin to focus your thoughts and start working through the checklist, the energies in the house will naturally begin to change. So, it is important that you deal with any spirits that may be there first as they will start to feel the changes of the energy, begin to feel uneasy and possibly agitated, that is when you may get some poltergeist activity.

Poltergeist purely means 'noisy spirit' in German. It is just a spirit or three that have become unsettled due to the changing atmosphere in the house. So, if you don't have the time to work through the whole of the checklist all in one go, do, please, make sure that you move the spirits into the light as soon as possible, ideally as soon as you have found out who they are, when they died and why. Finding out this information not only shows respect but makes it easier to help their transit to the light.

The same can be done for any attachments that you find on yourself and your family. Other than that, work through the checklist diligently, and follow the order of questions, as they have been arranged in order of importance.

## Animal Healing

Many of the healing techniques in this book can also be used to help animals. Like us, they can be subjected to curses and spells, can attract attachments (especially from their owners), suffer from emotional stress, have abandonment issues, or have a spirit or elementals attached to them and much more.

Keep your pets in mind, as you work through the checklist, and check them for each issue as you go. Their healing should be carried out in the same way as for you and your home.

Do also look at their stables, kennels or the location of their bed, as they may have detrimental lines running through them that will need to be worked on and healed to help them maintain or get back to full fitness.

## Before you begin, you will need:

Pendulum or rods

A range of fine tipped coloured pens

A ruler

Paper

Floorplan

A clipboard or heavy weight to hold the plan in place as you work on it.

A crystal wand/pointer

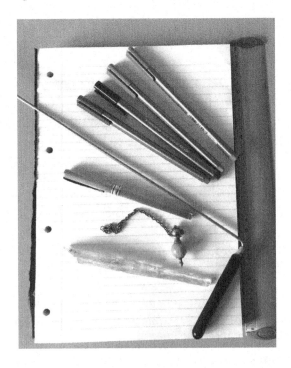

*You will need some basic tools*

Floorplans come in all shapes and sizes, and you do not necessarily need one that is to scale (but as close as it can possibly be is helpful), a hand-drawn one is also fine. It is best to have the plan clear of room descriptions and furniture, so you are left with just an outline of each room and the house itself. If you have an estate agent's plan or scale drawings, you could scan it and then clear any superfluous details that you do not need, as I have shown in the examples below:

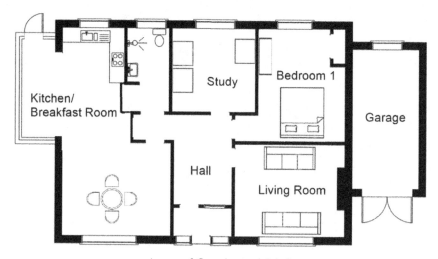

*A normal floorplan with labels*

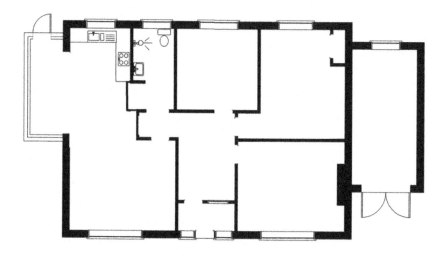

*A clear floorplan is much easier to work on with*

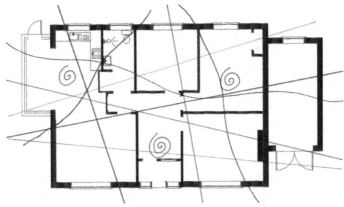

*An example of how your house plan may look after working through all the questions*

I only tend to work on the ground floor plan, but it's good to also have the upper floors of the house just in case there is an individual problem to be found in one of the rooms, like a sinkhole, portal or power artefact.

In most cases, the lines drawn on the ground floor tend to be echoed upstairs. I use different colours for different lines, you can create your own key and use what colours you have.

Working through each topic, dowsing the questions, obtaining the answers, and then drawing up your house plan will take time and it may take you several days or weeks to complete. However, as mentioned before, I do feel that it is important to carry out the full healing in one session.

The only one caveat to that statement is when you find any lost souls (spirits) in the house. I then (as already mentioned) recommend you deal with them straight away, helping them continue their journey to the light, as soon as possible

## Rating System

When I dowse, I use a simple rating system (as shown in the dowsing section), to explain how detrimental the various areas are in the house. Please do not forget that we are only looking for areas and lines that are harmful to the family, if they are not detrimental, leave them alone.

You can download a workbook from my website which includes this checklist and the related questions. (click on the shop, then the book cover and enter the word PENDULUM.)

# Heal your Home Checklist

## Spirits, Attachments, Human Manifested Energy Forms

1. Spirits, Ghosts, Tricky Spirits, Trapped Souls

1a. Spirits Attached to the Auric Field

2. Detrimental/Inappropriate Attachments

3. Detrimental Energy Forms (Human Manifested)

4. Lower Animal Life Forms

5. Sorcery/Black Magic

6. Spirit Lines

## Earth Energies

7. Water Veins/Underground Streams

8. Any other detrimental water source

9. Earth Energy Lines

10. Energy Channels

11. Fault Lines

12. Dynamic Energy Lines

13. Human Intent Lines

14. Energy Spirals

15. Energetic Sink Holes

16. Reversal Points

## Detrimental Human Energy Patterns

17. Emotional Energy Areas (Human Conflict)

18. Psychic Cords

19. Dimensional Portals

20. Illness Trigger Points

21. Consecrated Ground

22. Curses or Spells

23. Psychic Attack

24. Power Artefacts

25. Place Memory

26. Interdimensional Place Memory

27. Vows or Contracts

28. Fractured/Torn Souls

29. Stress/Disturbance Lines (Man-made)

30. Karmic Problems – Simultaneous Life Trauma

30a. Karmic Problems – Parallel Life Trauma

31. Detrimental Implants

32. Toxic Lines

33. Chakra Alignments and/or Blockages

34. Anything else affecting the house and family (in garden/ grounds or close by)

35. Fabric of the Building

36. Anaesthetic Traces, Inoculations, Vaccinations, Heavy Metals

37. Parasites

## Off-World Energies

## Technopathic Stress, Fracking

## Guardian Spirits, Elementals

## Detrimental Animal Energies

## Associated Healing

# 1. Spirits, Ghosts, Tricky Spirits, Trapped Souls

Whenever I carry out an investigation on a house, I will always start by finding out if there are any lost souls or discarnate beings present. They can be the source of many problems and need to be dealt with as soon as possible. If you plan to work through the whole checklist in one go and then carry out a healing straight afterwards, you can move the spirits through then. But if there is going to be a time delay of a few days or weeks then I suggest you stop, once you have found out the necessary information, and carry out a soul rescue. The longer you leave it the more chance there is of nightly disturbances.

They may be as unaware of you as you are of them, but as soon as you start changing any of the energetic patterns in the home, any resident spirit will be affected and start to feel uncomfortable. This is the time that you may get some poltergeist activity. This is not like you see in the movies, but you may get objects moving, strange noises and of course odd smells around the house.

Always treat these spirits or souls with the greatest of respect, as indeed you should with all the questions on the checklist. Do remember that no one likes to be forced or made to do anything, so it is always better, when conversing with them, to do so nicely and calmly. Just as we experience a big upheaval when we move home, a lost soul, as they move into the light, can feel the same way. Be gentle, understanding and aware of their feelings.

Over the years, I have found that every spirit who has not gone to the light will naturally give off a detrimental energy. It is not because they have ill-intentions towards you, it is simply because they should not have remained here in the form that they are now in. Do remember that a lost soul does not have to have lived and died in your home, or indeed have had any connection to you or it. They are often attracted by your energies, or those of your children, and can follow you home from the shops or work, then becoming an unwanted house guest.

Children can be an excellent indicator to there being a spirit in the house, as they are more open and perceptive to these energy patterns. Many are able to see lost souls or ghosts and even communicate with them. Because children's life energies are so vibrant, spirits can be attracted to their 'buzz', and can often become attached to them. Rather like surrogate grandparents, they care for them, look after them and can become fiercely protective of them too. Any parent that scolds the child who has a spirit close to them, needs to be careful, as they could be asking for trouble.

Often, trapped or lost souls want to move to the light, but they need help to do so, and therefore can attach themselves to anyone they believe can help. These lost souls do not, in most cases, mean to be a nuisance, frighten or harm anyone. However, they can get frustrated, particularly if ignored.

I have slightly changed the removal process of these spirits over the last few years, as I began to discover that a number of them were finding it difficult to move through. As I tuned into them, I found that they still had attachments (blobs of detrimental emotion) within their aura and both physical and psychic cords still linking them to family and friends that were, in effect, holding them back.

Once discovered, their attachments cleared and cords all cut, these lost souls can normally be easily moved on. This is not an exorcism; they are not being banished or sent off to bother someone else, but merely given another chance to go to the light, to move off the earth plane. I always ask for a vision of what awaits them to be shown, as this often speeds up the process. Talk to them; they will listen to you and, in most cases, happily go on their travels.

You will sometimes find a 'tricky spirit', one who will not move on due to the uncertainty of what awaits them, perhaps fearing retribution for what they have done whilst alive. They may just enjoy the atmosphere of the house and the energy of the family, or, possibly, enjoy causing upset and mayhem. Some spirits can also attach themselves to people and start to control them.

So, the more information that you can find out about the spirit, and, potentially, why they are fearful or reticent about going to the light, the easier it should be to help them move them through. In basic terms you are showing that paradise awaits them, who wouldn't want to go?

Dowse all the questions with your rods or pendulum making detailed notes as you go. The following case studies should help show you the way.

## Case Study: A Village in Scotland

I received a telephone call from a healer called Heather, asking if I could remove an 'evil spirit' from her home that was affecting her and her animals. It sounded like a straightforward job, so I said yes. Little did I know what awaited me, and how long it would take to sort out the problems that they were experiencing.

It turned out that Heather and her sister Meg were both talented natural healers, regularly dowsing remedies for themselves and their animals. As I worked through the initial problem it became apparent that it wasn't just one spirit that needed moving on, but a whole host of them, plus a lot of nasty energy left behind by a jealous and controlling ex-husband who had passed over some years before.

In the past, they had called upon other people to work on the problems, but the healers had either given up or found that they just could not help. For several days, I was moving spirits into the light, but no sooner had one or two gone, they were replaced by more. I cleared and regularly closed all the doorways that had been opened by Heather and Meg during their healings, but these stretched back almost 30 years, so a lot had to be dealt with. I also performed some land healing, as the fields surrounding Heather's home were used by the Army as training grounds during World War II. I helped all the lost souls that had any connection to the old base to travel to the light irrespective of where they may now be, I also helped any that were stuck at the location.

Despite this, still more arrived and I continued to help moving them through. Heather's conservatory seemed to be a popular place for them to congregate, so that was regularly cleared too, and then sealed and protected to stop further influx.

Their pets and animals were also being psychically attacked, which, I was told by Upstairs, was on the harmful and express instructions left behind by Meg's late husband, whose energy remained around the sisters. Once he had been moved into the light, his influences waned and are thankfully were no more. There were also E.T. problems, attachments affecting both sisters, detrimental human created thought forms, trapped nature spirits and so on. It was a wonder they were both as healthy as they were.

There were many layers of problems to work through, some were human created, and these had combined with lost souls to form a very complex web that was slow to unravel, and I had to peel back many, many layers to reach a satisfactory conclusion. Then there were the memories to clear. They had lived with all of these detrimental energies for such a long time, almost 50 years, and the upset, pain and fear was lodged deeply in their subconscious minds, which can be difficult to clear by the person affected, so healing was needed.

I worked at cellular level, clearing away the stored memories, then sending healing to the physical body, the mental and finally the spiritual. I paid special attention to the pineal gland and the reptilian brain, as they both needed serious clearing. Having lived with these problems every day for all those years, it almost became a way of life. The spirit interference, from the past, was expected, and didn't fail to deliver.

Like many natural healers, neither Heather nor Meg had realised, or known, that once you have finished a healing session, or even a simple dowsing exercise, you must not only close yourself down, clearing away any detrimental energy patterns that might have been created, but equally as important, is to ensure that all doorways that might have been opened during the session, whether expectedly or unexpectedly are firmly closed.

Leaving all the doorways open each time, enabled hundreds of spirits to gather over the fifty years, meaning that there were untold layers of them to move into the light.

This took many months to solve. After several hundred lost souls were moved to the light, the last pieces of the puzzle were gradually falling into place. The controlling late ex-husband and all the instructions that he had left behind were finally cleared and the number of spirits appearing gradually dwindled until we reached the final few. It then got down to removing one lost soul at a time until the final spirit was helped through. The last one was the most powerful and needed special treatment.

During the final edit of this book, in January 2021, I was contacted again by Meg, and further healing needed to be carried out. Other problems had arisen, and this involved what can only be described as circles or bands of energy that were affecting Meg and her animals. The detrimental thoughts of her sister's ex-husband had mutated in an extraordinary way.

The vision that I received was just like a snake eating its own tail, an endless circle. There were several that had been created and in a number of different dimensions, so some head scratching went on before I worked out how to clear them.

Once I felt I had found the solution, (after dowsing the possibilities) I asked my guides and archangels to help me deal with them. I simply asked that they be prised apart, manipulated, and stretched into a straight line, and as this happened, they shattered into small pieces and these were then taken to the light and disposed of appropriately.

This has been a very complex case, and although we have nearly reached the conclusion, the spirits are still appearing intermittently. I believe that there is one underlying spirit that will only be reached once all the layers above her are removed. She is an unhappy soul and does need to go to the light to continue her destiny. But she will only go when the time is appropriate.

Keep in mind, as you diagnose the problems in your home, and perform a healing, to regularly check on the family members. It is possible that, when moving on a lost soul, one might, at some stage, decide not to go and attach themselves to a member of the family. This is a rare occurrence, but I think it's better to be forewarned.

When carrying out any form of healing you need to ask the question 'Are there any more spirits for me to deal with?' If the answer comes back as yes, then you will need, at some stage, to go through the process again to move them through. This may be over the next few days, in a week or so's time or several months later. I always check to find out the best time to move the next layer of spirits on and then put a note in my diary. It can take many years for the energy patterns to become so deep and dark, therefore healing is not always an overnight success and therefore needs careful managing.

You should be able to move all the lost souls through, into the light, in one go. But sometimes you will find that one wishes to be treated individually. As I have already mentioned, I like to find out as much information about them as I can, before I move them through, it shows respect. But I understand that it might not be easy, especially as you are just starting out, to do so. The Universe is very forgiving, try your best and they will help you. If you have five or more in your home, they will normally go en masse without you needing to dig too deeply into their history.

## *Dowsing diagnostic questions for spirits, ghosts, tricky spirits, trapped souls:*

1. How many spirits are there in the home?
2. How detrimental each one is to me and the family?
3. Is there a main spirit I need to know more about?
4. When did they pass away?
5. How old were they when they passed away?
6. How did they pass away?
7. Do they have any attachments that need to be cleared?
8. Are there any cords that are keeping them here?
9. Are any of them tricky souls?
10. Where are they?
11. Are they all happy to go to the light today?
12. Is there another layer of spirits to move on?
13. Are there any spirits in the car(s) or outbuildings?
14. Is there anything else that I need to know?

# *1a. Spirits Attached to the Auric Field*

Spirits in the auric field are very different to what I would call attachments, which, to me, are black blobs of energy made up of detrimental human emotion. Spirits that are attached to the auric field are lost souls that have been attracted to a person, have entered their auric field, and then become an influencing factor in their life.

In most cases, our aura is too strong to allow spirits to attach, but any form of trauma, illness, stress, or unhappiness can weaken these protective bands surrounding our body and potentially let a lost soul in. Once attached, they can be difficult to move on, and they can become an integral part of the affected person.

This can bring profound changes to the person affected. They may experience shortness of temper and irritability, altered personality, constant headaches, cravings for certain types of food, spasmodic body movements, facial tics, insomnia, nightmares and even their eyes may change colour.

The affected person may not notice that anything is wrong, although this is not always the case. They may experience constant chattering voices in their head, yearn for sugar-based food, a feeling of never being alone, insomnia, and even start to wear or style their hair in a different way to mimic the attached spirit.

One of the questions that I ask (no. 8 in the diagnostic questions) is 'Why and when did they attach'? Sometimes it can be because a spirit simply liked the person's energy, or it can be a deeper attraction (like a young man espying a pretty woman), or perhaps a spirit wanting to protect a particular person (a mother wanting to look after a young toddler), or just a mischievous spirit wanting to cause problems.

1a

Knowing when the spirit attached can help us to identify the weakness in the person's auric field (our natural shield). This can be through drug or alcohol abuse, depression, physical and mental trauma or injury, times of high stress levels and so on. Often finding out the month and year can help pinpoint why our defence mechanism had been weakened to such an extent that it allowed an energetic presence to attach to us.

This information then helps us in the healing process, as we can then pay special attention to healing what caused the weakness and strengthen the aura to ensure that no further spirits can get through. This is why I stress how important daily psychic protection is.

## Case Study: Injury Trauma

A mother called me about her teenage son called Robin. She didn't know what the problem was, but she knew that something wasn't right. Robin had been a sporty lad at school, but had badly injured his ankle whilst playing rugby, meaning a short spell in hospital. Before the injury, he had been an open and communicative lad, full of fun and well liked at his boarding school.

After the injury, he had become very withdrawn and was spending a lot of time, at home, in his bedroom which was becoming like a cave. He did not want to go out and in his mother's, words had become 'a right slob'. She felt that he was developing ADHD, so she spoke to her local GP who wanted to put him on a dose of anti-depressants.

She asked me to carry out a full house and family healing, and during my investigative work I picked up that Robin actually had a female spirit attached to him and it was she, I felt, who was causing the problems/ personality change. The spirit was very possessive and didn't want him mixing with others. She was jealous of his friends, and his family, and was the cause of him slowly withdrawing from the world.

She had passed away in 1904 aged 13 due to a bad case of the mumps. She had been attached to another man for many years until he had passed away, in the same hospital that Robin had been admitted to. As the old man died, she detached herself, was attracted by Robin's youthful energy and linked straight into him, slotting into his aura that was already weak from the injury trauma, just like a piece from a jigsaw puzzle.

Once I found her, it was not difficult to move her into the light, by showing her a vision of what awaited her. I did throw out a small threat, saying that if she did not go straight away and willingly, I would keep working on Robin and she would have no respite. Although I always recommend remaining calm and being gentle with spirits, sometimes, you have to tell it like it is.

I called Robin's mother and told her that the spirit had now gone, and her words made me smile and feel very humble at the same time: 'Robin came downstairs about 11.30, he was grinning and had the same look on his face as he does when he comes back to us after a term at school, almost as though he was seeing everything afresh. He had showered and dressed in clean clothes, brought his dirty washing down with him and put it in the machine. He came over to me and gave me a big hug, sat down and ate a huge breakfast. We had our boy back'.

Now, not every case will produce such speedy and noticeable results, and this one was quite unusual. It can take days, or sometimes weeks to see the changes, but if a spirit is the problem then by removing it, there will certainly be beneficial effects, not just for the person affected but for the whole family.

## Mental Health Issues

Keeping our auras and bodies clear of unwanted guests and attachments can greatly help our mental health. We are all affected, to a certain extent, by other people's emotions, moods, and thoughts, as well as the stresses and strains of modern-day life. And it's no different to being affected by spirits and entities.

Spiritual Hygiene is therefore very important. By clearing and protecting yourself each morning, it helps you to be yourself. Keeping your mind, body and soul free of outside interference (from people in this realm and

90

in others) will bring you clarity, enabling you to see and think clearly without the baggage that most of us carry around.

**NB** It is important that if you are at all worried about yourself or any member of your family, you seek help from a medical professional but do keep an open mind when it comes to complementary therapies.

## *Dowsing diagnostic questions for spirits attached to the auric field:*

1.  Does (name) have any spirits attached to his/her aura?

2.  How detrimental are they (0 to -10)?

3.  When did they attach to (name)?

4.  Are they male or female?

5.  When did they pass over?

6.  What age where they when they passed?

7.  What caused them to die (Natural causes, unnatural, disease)?

8.  Why and when did they attach to (name)?

9.  Can I remove them today and help them into the light?

10. If not today, then when? (tomorrow, next week?)

11. Will they go easily or there anything else I need to know?

12. Do I need someone else's help to remove them and send them to the light?

13. If so, who? (Family member, friend, healer, archangel, spirit guide or protector)

14. Is there a good time to carry out the removal ceremony? If so, when?

# 2. Detrimental/Inappropriate Attachments

These attachments are 'black blobs of detrimental energy', caused by fear, stress, unhappiness, uncertainty, arguments, illness and worry. Any angry outbursts – which releases detrimental energy – will cause an attachment to form.

This can then join to another detrimental 'black blob', gaining in strength. The stronger they become the easier it is for them to attach themselves to you or another human being, either within your auric field or, worse still, linked to one of your chakras.

They are like the sticky buds you find when out walking in the countryside. It doesn't matter how much you try to avoid them, there is always one adhering to you somewhere.

These attachments will feed off your energy, leaving you feeling drained, both physically and mentally. If they stay attached for a long time, mental and emotional problems can form, easily leading to depression and illness.

Just as I detailed in the case study on spirits linking into your auric field; hospitals, in particular, are places where attachments are created due to the trauma, illness, injuries and emotional stress and upset. The heavy noxious atmosphere can also make it easier for these detrimental emotional energy patterns to attach to you as you are probably in an anxious state yourself.

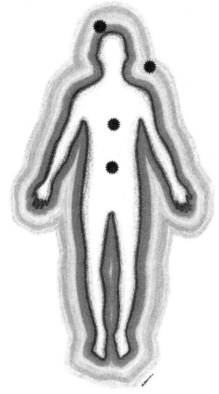

*Figure showing attachments to the aura and body*

So, if you are going to hospital for a check-up, an operation, or are just visiting, please make sure that you are fully protected psychically by employing the psychic protection method, you can also carry out this exercise for the person that you are visiting, to help keep them safe and free of attachments.

All attachments need to be moved on as soon as they are detected, the longer they are with you, the worse you are going to feel and the longer it will take for the effects to wear off.

I spend a lot of my time when working on a family removing these little nasties. In my courses I do say that although they can influence us, they won't, or can't, turn a normally placid person into an axe murderer, but they will play havoc with their emotions. The depth of their detrimental effect will, of course, depend on the mental health of the person that they are affecting.

If you work in the health sector (Therapist, Masseur, Reiki Healer, Nurse, Doctor etc.) I would suggest that you check your body and aura for attachments at least once a day, especially after working closely on or with a client/patient. I would say the same to those who regularly commute to work, surrounded by people with emotional baggage, some of which will undoubtedly stick to you.

Hairdressers also need to be very careful as they are not only working within a client's etheric field (the closest to the body), but also working on the physical body. It is, therefore, so much easier for attachments to move across, and they undoubtedly will.

## Dowsing diagnostic questions for detrimental/ inappropriate attachments:

1. How many attachments does each member of the family have?
2. How detrimental are they to each member on a scale from 0 to -10?
3. When did they attach?
4. Why did they attach? (During depression, stress, relationship, trauma?)
5. Can they easily be removed?
6. Can I remove them?
7. If I cannot remove them, can someone else?
8. Is there anything else that I need to know?
9. How many have I created over the years?
10. Can I carry out a healing and clear them all?
11. Is psychic protection the answer to keep me clear?

# 3. Detrimental Energy Forms (Human Manifested)

Previously called Human Manifested Energy Forms, most of them (life forms and thought forms) have come into existence during Global Conflicts, the First and Second World wars in particular. They are formed by the combined emotions of hundreds, if not thousands or millions, of people.

In essence both a thought form and life form are created in the same way, from conflict. But there is a subtle difference between the two. A thought form comes mainly from mental upset, internal anxiety, stress, and illness. Whereas a life form is mostly created by people unhappy with their living and working conditions, feeling stuck in a rut and going nowhere, the effect of abuse and so on.

The horrors of the war, hatred of the opposing sides, fear that we may lose, sadness and grief over the dead, uncertainty at what life might be like when the conflict is over and worry for loved ones involved in the fighting, all blend together to create these detrimental forms.

If you are visiting a site that is linked to a war, then it's even more important to ensure you are fully protected, so that you don't attract the attention of one of these detrimental energy forms. They are strong enough to survive as a free-floating form, without being attached to either a person or their aura. You may just be the unlucky individual whose energy pattern is attractive to them and end up taking them home.

They are the black shadows that you often see out of the corner of your eye, and as you turn around, they have disappeared. This is to do with the rod cells (photoreceptors) in your eyes. If you look directly at something it vanishes, yet if you look slightly to one side it reappears. People often say they have seen a ghost, but I think it is more than likely to have been a thought or life Form.

Though they are not particularly commonplace, it is worth checking your home to make sure that you do not have one of these dark beings lurking around.

These energy forms are also created by repeated arguments and detrimental thoughts, and so 'divorce houses' (homes where the occupants move in, divorce and move out) will more than likely have one or more of these human manifested forms in residence, creating, influencing, and causing further conflict between the warring couple.

## Case Study: Covid-19

The global fear and worry caused by Covid-19 spawned a new generation of these detrimental forms. I found my first one in June 2020 and removed it from a client's home. The family lived in constant panic and consternation over catching the Covid-19 virus. They admitted that they were avidly watching the news on the television and were feeling worse each day as the numbers of those affected increased.

This is the perfect scenario for the entrance of a thought form. Emotions deepened, all members of the family had become very irritable and tempers regularly flared. It was a very unhappy household. They called me and asked me to do a full house healing, but I didn't feel that was necessary, and after asking a few pertinent questions I found the thought form that had been created by their concern, that had also been added to by the collective global fear, and quickly sent it into the light.

They reported back to me a few days later to say that they all felt so much better, the house had a calmer atmosphere and felt lighter and brighter.

Since then, I have found many more of these thought forms created by the anxiety, uncertainty, fear etc of many hundreds, if not thousands of people. Not only the worries of contracting the virus but also their concerns over the possible detrimental affects of the vaccine.

## *Dowsing diagnostic questions for detrimental energy forms:*

1. Are there any detrimental energy forms in the house?
2. How many are there?
3. How detrimental are they?
4. Are they thought forms or life forms?
5. How long have they been in existence?
6. How long have they been in the house?
7. Why are they in the home?
8. Are they easily moved on?
9. Is there anything else that I need to know before I move them on?

3

# 4. Lower Animal Life Forms

These lower animal life forms have lived on this planet, but they come from a time before humans existed. They do have form, but this is mainly an energetic outline (rather like an aura) than a physical one. When man first arrived on Earth, we did not have the full range of emotions that we do today, therefore these lower life forms find this rather unique aspect of us fascinating and that is why they attach themselves to us.

Because they are unemotional, they like to experience how we human beings function emotionally. They love the roller coaster ride of what we call life. The more emotional the person, the more they like it. They can influence, in a modest way, how we react to given situations and problems.

They are mostly found within our auric fields. However, they can sometimes become attached to our chakras. You will need to check where they are when dowsing. They need to be carefully removed making sure, above all, that they leave nothing behind - this includes their seeds and tentacles.

Interestingly, I have never found them attached to anyone with autism or any form of mental illness, such as Alzheimer's.

You don't need to know too much information about them, simply where they are, how many there are and when they attached, and you can then use the simple method in the healing section to remove them.

## Dowsing diagnostic questions for lower animal life forms:

1. Are there any lower animal life forms connected to anyone in the family?

2. How many does each member of the family have attached?

3. How detrimental are they?

4. When did they attach?

5. Why are they here? (To learn about human behaviour etc.)

6. Are they easily removed?

7. Is there anything else that I need to know (before I remove them)?

4

# 5. Sorcery/Black Magic

I have added the word 'sorcery' to this title, as I feel that it can better describe some of the problems that we need to look for when we are dowsing our home.

Black magic has very dark connotations and it will be a rare occurrence for you to come across it in your own home. Unless of course, someone has been messing around with a Ouija board, are actively delving into mystical ceremonies, have inherited it from past occupiers or been playing a particularly bizarre or supernatural game on their X-Box or PlayStation.

I have found that some computer games can be responsible for the creation and opening of black magic portals. The games can be totally absorbing when you play them, and depending on the subject, can affect your subconscious mind. I found this exact problem in a client's house on the south coast of England.

## Case Study – X-Box

A mother contacted me, concerned that her youngest son was always in a dark mood and slowly withdrawing from the family. He was spending more and more time in his bedroom playing games on his X-Box. It appeared that the games were almost controlling him, not the other way round. His eyes had also changed colour. According to his mother, they were getting dark and lifeless.

I picked up that he was being detrimentally affected by a computer game and called his mother to discuss what I had found. She knew straight away which game it was and told me that he was obsessed with it. I had already identified which game it was, telling her where, in the bedroom it was located, and also identifying which shelf it was on (counting in from the right-hand side which DVD sleeve contained the actual disc). It matched the game that she suspected, and she quickly dispatched the disc and cover into the wheelie bin. I performed a clearing on it just in case someone else found the game and started playing it.

Once the problem had been diagnosed and the game was disposed of, I got to work on the son and his room, including the X-Box. First, I had to gather together all the detrimental energies that had come through, and return them, via the doorway that had been created, to another dimension. Once done, I made sure that the doorway was closed and then cleared away any further energetic patterns that had been created (mostly around the bed where he lay to play the game). I cleared the X-Box and filled the room with divine white light, leaving it in peace, balance and harmony.

I then worked on the son, making sure that he was clear of all attachments, and anything else that had been affecting him detrimentally, sending him protection to make sure he was no longer vulnerable or open to further attack. I asked the mother to give me an update in a few days' time to make sure that all was well with her son. She told me that he was much happier, had stopped having nightmares, was sleeping well, he had begun to smile again, and his dark moods had totally disappeared.

It would be a good idea for us to be more aware of what effects computer games can have on our children, and some horror films or TV shows too. As you watch them at home, doorways can open through the TV or computer screen, allowing detrimental energies in. The same can also happen at a cinema, which can be even more hazardous, as you have all the energies of other people's emotional states and fear that can feed whatever arrives and make it stronger too.

I stopped watching horror films after I watched The Exorcist when it was first released., It scared the bejesus out of me, I then had a thirty-minute ride home in the dark on my very underpowered motorbike. Every tree came alive, the shadows moved, and I wasn't a happy bunny, I can tell you.

Sorcery is the use of magic, and in particular, black magic. It can mean the use of evil spirits when divining, casting spells and curses. When I ask the question, as I work on a clients home, I use it in a wider sense, so that it covers a multitude magical energy patterns. Witchcraft is also looked for when I dowse for sorcery.

There are men and women who have used their knowledge and energy to cause people harm, and traces of this sorcery can linger for some time. I have had to deal with several cases over the years, mainly in older houses dating back to medieval times. A coven would often gather in secret, for fear of discovery by the authorities or church, and carry out their secret ceremonies. These detrimental energy patterns could still adversely affect anyone living there today.

Be careful to only ask to find the detrimental patterns in the house, as many of the witches that I know today are healers, theirs is an ancient, almost Shamanistic way, a timeless practice using natural herbs, well-practiced spells, working for the good of the people using ceremonies that have been repeated many times over the years. These acts of magic will not be detrimental to the occupants and can be left alone.

## Case Study – Threefold Law

I was called upon to investigate an old house, which had a timbered dining room with a spectacular Inglenook fireplace that was rarely used. No one in the family liked the room and was mainly reserved for Christmas get-togethers. When I work on a house, I don't like to be given too much information, as I prefer to carry out my investigations with nothing to influence my findings

I found that the room had been used for sinister purposes in the distant past. Witches had met here, to send their combined thoughts out to harm others. Not innocent people, but those who had harmed others. The threefold law perhaps, though actioned purposefully. In Wicca it is believed that everything you do and send out into the world, will come back to you threefold, the good and bad. Some were farmers stealing land, some had badly treated their workers, others were cattle thieves, and the clergy were also targeted. This seems to have gone on for many years and had left an indelible imprint in the room.

There were a number of layers to remove, as you can imagine. I started with the first one, using light and love to clear it, and then waited until the next layer rose to the surface and then dealt with that. It took several weeks, but we got to the bottom of the problem eventually.

There were also a lot of energy lines running beneath the house, a number of water veins, which were all worked on as a matter of course. The client who called me in was the mother of the family, but she hadn't told her children about the house healing work that was being carried out, as she wanted to see what how they would react without knowing.

After weeks of clearing and healing, she came home one day to find her three teenagers sitting in the dining room, with a fire going, happily playing Monopoly.

## *Dowsing diagnostic questions for sorcery/black magic:*

1. Has black magic been practiced in this house?
2. Has any form of sorcery been practiced in this house?
3. Has any form of witchcraft been practised in this house?
4. Where did it take place?
5. Is there a detrimental area that needs healing?
6. Is it detrimental to me or my family?
7. If it is, how detrimental is it (0 to -10)?
8. Can I clear it myself using the healing method in this book?
9. If not, do I need to enlist the help of a friend to increase the healing energies? Who?

# 6. Spirit Lines

For the next few questions on the checklist, it is a good idea to chart them on the plan of your home. As I have already mentioned the drawing does not need to be 100% accurate or to scale, as long as it closely represents the layout of the house.

See '*Before You Begin, You Will Need*' in Part Two – Preparation, for more in-depth details on house plan requirements.

A spirit line is a pathway that spirits use on a regular basis, it may be very familiar to them as they could possibly have walked it when they were alive.

Even though houses may have been built over these pathways or lines, spirits will continue to use them instinctively. There can be just a few spirits, or many hundreds, depending on where you live. I don't necessarily find that these lines are harmful, although they can be. They can distressing for the people whose homes are affected by them and, of course, their pets. They may sometimes have a detrimental charge attached; it really does depend on what events happened on the line to make it so.

When you work on the line it is good to help as many lost souls go to the light as possible, then check to see if any have been left behind. Some may have been hesitant and not wanting to move through en masse, so be sure to look out for any stragglers and then help them move on, then double check to make sure they have all been dealt with effectively.

Ask to see whether there may be any further lost souls to move through in the future, then carry out a cleansing of the line, as detailed in the healing section.

When I find a spirit line, I normally mark it in purple on the house plan.

## Dowsing diagnostic questions for spirit lines:

1. Is there a spirit line affecting the home?
2. How many are there?
3. How detrimental is each line (if more than one)?
4. How many spirits use it?
5. How long is it?
6. How long has it been in existence?
7. Can all the spirits be moved into the light?
8. Will they all go at the same time (if not then find out when you can do the clearing)?
9. Is the line now fully healed?

6

# 7. Water Veins/ Underground Streams

Locating and dealing with the detrimental effects of water veins is a very important part of geomancy (earth healing), as they can be a major factor of geopathic stress and are known to be the root cause of many illnesses, including rheumatism, arthritis, and even cancer. The crossing points of these rivulets of water running beneath your home can be particularly detrimental, often as high as -10.

Having your bed situated above or near a crossing point of water veins can be particularly harmful, because your body relaxes during sleep, so it becomes more vulnerable to these detrimental external energies. A deep uninterrupted sleep is so important, as that is when the body repairs and heals itself from the stress and rigours of the day.

Symptoms of water veins beneath your bed can show themselves as disturbed sleep patterns, night sweats, bad dreams and feeling more tired upon awaking than when you went to bed.

It is also essential to sleep in a dark bedroom (ideally with blackout curtains) to help your pineal gland generate melatonin, the sleep hormone, because this helps regulate your sleep patterns. You can buy melatonin as a supplement, but it is far better for the body to generate it naturally.

In *Heal Your Home*, I wrote about water holding emotion, and science has now confirmed that it does hold memory, good and bad. Therefore, you not only have the energetic movement of the water causing you problems but also the possible memories of thousands of people flowing beneath your home contained within the molecules.

Also, do not forget that each drop of water you consume is millions of years old and therefore it not only contains the memory patterns of the dinosaurs but all those millions of people who have already been in contact with it. Water, like energy, never disappears, it is simply recycled.

When dowsing and tracing these water veins on a client's plan and producing the report, I only used to include one measurement when detailing how far the detrimental effects could be felt from the centre of the water vein. I have now added to this and like to ascertain not just how far to either side these noxious energies can be felt but also now how far above.

The reason? It is what I call the chimney effect, the detrimental energies can, in many cases, rise higher above the water veins than they do either side.

Working on, moving and healing the water veins can have a remarkable effect on people, their homes and animals; you are effectively removing all the detrimental emotion contained within them, clearing away any noxious earth energy patterns as well anything else that might be affecting you and your family.

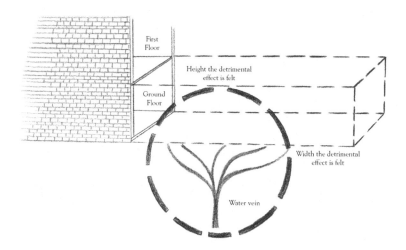

*The detrimental effects of a water vein beneath the house*

## Dowsing diagnostic questions for water veins/underground streams:

1. Are there any water veins affecting the home?

2. How many?

3. Where are they? (mark them as a line on the house plan in blue)

4. How detrimental are they (0 to -10)?

5. How far to either side (width) and above (height) can the detrimental effects of the water veins be felt?

6. How deep are they beneath the ground?

7. How much of the detrimental energy coming from it is human emotion?

8. Can I heal the whole water vein?

9. Can I divert them all from underneath my house?

10. Can I divert them away from other houses that they affect (always ask if appropriate)?

7

# 8. Any other detrimental water source

Water veins are only a small part of a larger problem. There can be many other water related issues in the home that need to be dealt with, hence the reason for the separate question.

To start with we will be looking at blindhead springs, or water domes which are a naturally occurring phenomena. If you are unlucky to have one rising beneath your home, you will probably experience similar problems to the crossing points of water veins.

Water is being forced upwards from many miles beneath the earth, and it rises freely until it hits an impermeable layer of rock or clay, the water then spreads out into many smaller rivulets. However, the energy generated on its journey continues to move upwards through the earth and into your home, affecting all the floors above.

The detrimental energies produced can spread anywhere from a few feet in width to several yards which could incorporate the whole of your house. The detrimental effects of living above a blindhead spring can include the following: feelings of vertigo, insomnia, lack of energy and nausea, it can be likened to being trapped in a whirlpool of energy.

This energy has been harnessed by humans over the years, and they can often be found rising beneath the altar in a church, for instance. This gives the holiest place in a church a special feel or buzz. An energy spiral is often present too, formed by the swirling energies of the rising water.

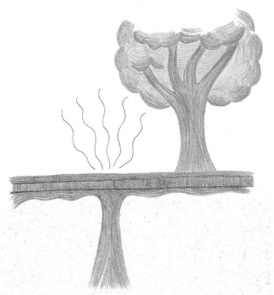

*A blindhead spring underground, and the reach of the detrimental energies*

These blindhead springs are also thought to play their part in the formation of crop circles. Not the intricate ones, many of those are man-made, but the smaller rudimentary circles. A combination of rising water connecting with the air above to create a small whirlwind or vortex that flattens the corn (or other such crops) to create an almost perfect but rough circle. So, you can imagine the effect that would have on a sleeping body.

Along with these springs, we need to consider the energy of trapped ancient water. This is something that was brought to my attention by Neal Hawkins of Meridian Soils, a soil research engineering company, on a course that I was teaching in Essex. I first met him while I was giving a talk in Maldon. His sister, Jean, had dragged him along, since then though he has taken to house healing and dowsing like a duck to water (sorry). During one of my courses, I was describing how detrimental underground water can be and how it affects people, in particular water veins and blindhead springs, when Neal asked if water, trapped in clay, beneath someone's home could also be harmful?

It was not something that I had ever thought about, so I checked in with Upstairs and got a big 'yes'. Neil explained that during his soil and land surveys he often came across water that had been trapped for thousands, if not millions, of years, often in clay but other materials can also be involved. Since then, I have found several cases of ancient, trapped water affecting client's homes.

Everything has a vibrational energy and trapped water is no exception. But not all trapped ancient water will be detrimental, so when we are diagnosing our homes, we want to find what is harmful to us and our family. If it isn't damaging to the health of the occupants, leave it well alone. There is no harm in sending healing to these neutral pockets of water if you wish, but it will be definitely needed for the toxic ones.

When I dowse the question of whether the house or family is affected by trapped or ancient water and get a positive reaction, I look to find the central point or epicentre of the problem. I mark that on the house plan and by running my crystal pointer (a finger is just as good) away from the centre I ask to be shown the extent of the detrimental energy, wait until my rod or pendulum moves, and make a mark. Do the same on the opposite side of the central point and making another mark, keep going until you have mapped out the entire shape of the underground water. It may only be a few inches across (on the plan) or it may affect the whole of the house.

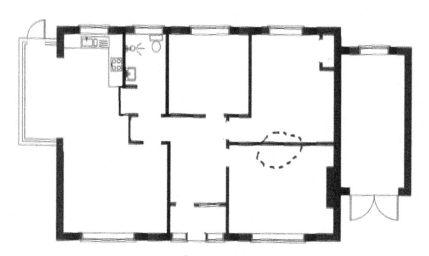

*A blindhead spring marked on the floorplan*

I feel that mapping these areas out shows respect to the problem, and by showing this respect you are part way to completing the healing.

The land use will have changed over thousands of years and we don't know what our garden was used for, say, back in the 1100s. Throughout history, water was worshipped, and it played its part in religious ceremonies, especially in pagan and druid rituals.

Springs, for instance, were viewed as magical, their waters never running dry, spouting directly from the sacred Earth, giving sustenance to people as well as irrigating their crops. The springs became consecrated by the repetition of the ceremonies performed, and the holy water was held in the highest esteem. Some springs were known to provide cures for blindness, infertility, the plague, rickets and other maladies.

Some springs are now dry at certain times of the year, or have just stopped altogether, but despite this, the area surrounding the spring would still have retained its sacredness. Then along came a builder, who has erected a house over the top and the family who then live in the home are wondering why they are having problems. The energies generated would be just like those underneath the altar of a church, vibrating at a higher level than is good for day to day living.

Capped wells (in houses) can also present a problem to health, but this is rare, because in most cases the water is still flowing and not static. If you know that you have a well either under the house or in the garden, regularly send it your blessings, they in turn will travel many miles underground, in the water, helping people, nature spirits and the land as it wends its way across the countryside. You could even dress the well once a year, with flowers and offerings. This is a regular occurrence in both Derbyshire and the Malverns. Water is sacred and do not forget that each drop is not just precious, but as I mentioned before, it is millions of years old.

## Dowsing diagnostic questions for other detrimental water sources:

1. Are there any other water sources that are detrimental to my family and house?

2. If so, is it a blindhead spring?

3. Trapped water?

4. Ancient water?

5. Is there a well that needs healing?

6. Is our home built above or near a sacred water site, that is affecting us detrimentally?

7. How detrimental is it to the family? (0 to -10)

8. Is there more than one layer of detrimental energy to heal?

8

# 9. Earth Energy Lines

Earth energy lines are the big power bands of the Earth, necessary for life to exist on the planet. Each one stretches around the planet, taking energy to where it is needed. They tend to run on or close to the surface of the planet and will expand and contract with human consciousness.

When working with these earthly lines, I draw them in as straight lines on a house floorplan in green. As with the water veins, I have started to include not just how far the detrimental energies affect you width wise, from the centre of the energy line, but also how far above. The chimney effect again.

Again, as with the water veins, these lines can also carry a certain amount of energetic human emotion within them and so I then dowse to see how much and how detrimental it is to the family.

These energy lines run around the globe, and you can imagine how many houses and businesses they intersect and interact with, millions probably. Each human within these buildings will be releasing their emotions, whether from stress, worry, exhaustion, upsets and so on, and these emotions become part of the line's molecular make up. Not all of it will be detrimental of course, there will be good vibrations too, for example, the line might run through a warm sandy beach in Greece where people are enjoying themselves.

When it comes to healing the earth energy line, if it's appropriate, I do a healing on the whole line surrounding the globe, not just the part that goes under the house. I often imagine the line running through an area of conflict and, as the healing happens, a peaceful thought goes through the minds of the people there.

Do not forget that when healing is carried out appropriately, it doesn't matter what you want or ask for, if the 'Highest of the High' doesn't want change or healing given, then it won't happen. However, never forget the power of negotiation, if the line is not healed the first time, always ask for a second time, or even a third. Or ask why it cannot be healed at this time, perhaps it can be at a later date.

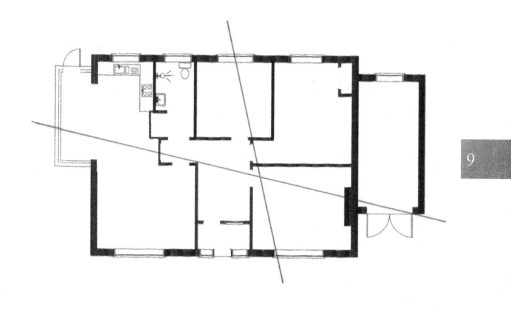

*Earth energy lines on a floorplan*

I recommend sending healing through the line to deal with the detrimental human emotion first, then finally clearing away any of the detrimental earth energies that might be left.

## Dowsing diagnostic questions for earth energy lines:

1. Are there any detrimental earth energy lines running through the home?

2. How many?

3. Where are they?

4. How detrimental are they?

5. How far to either side and above can the detrimental energies be felt?

6. Am I allowed to heal the whole line?

7. Will it stay healed or is there another layer to deal with? (If yes, then go to next question)

8. When will I have to deal with it? (Then find out when and put that date in your diary)

9. How much of the detrimental energy is made up of human emotion that needs clearing?

10. How much is made up of detrimental earth energy?

# 10. Energy Channels

These channels are a major part of the energy system of our planet. They weave around the world, feeding the main ley lines that they are associated with. Their contorted travels are often difficult to trace as they can react to human consciousness and move at will. They will certainly be found running through most, if not all, the sacred sites worldwide.

The large Michael Ley has probably the best-known energy channels (The Michael and Mary Lines) in the world associated with it, first mooted by John Michell (*A New View Over Atlantis*) and then famously tracked by Hamish Miller and Paul Broadhurst who then wrote a remarkable book called *The Sun and Serpent*, which is a must-read for anyone interested in earth energies.

The main Michael Ley, along which the rising sun travels on or near Mayday, runs from Carn Les Boel in Cornwall, before finally disappearing into the North Sea at Hopton-on-Sea in Norfolk.

The Michael and Mary lines are what I refer to as energy channels, they twist and turn on an almost serpentine-like path, feeding and interacting with the Michael Ley. On their journey, they pass through many sacred and holy sites including St. Michaels Mount, The Hurlers, Brentor Church, through the Church of the Holy Cross in Crediton, Cadbury Castle, Glastonbury and the Tor, Oliver's Castle near Devizes, Windmill Hill and the Henge at Avebury, the Abbey at Bury St. Edmund and on to Hopton-on-Sea.

The above is not an exhaustive list of where they flow through but shows how these amazing and intricate lines interact with and are utilised by us human beings. The big question is, which came first, the sacred site or the Michael and Mary lines. Was it the sacred or holy site, built by man, that attracted them or were their crossing points noted and monuments, such as Avebury Henge, then constructed above them?

Energy channels and leys can be found over the whole of the British Isles, and I am currently plotting a number of energy channels running through many of North Yorkshire's sacred sites. I hope to produce a book about them in the near future.

Purely out of interest, I remember dowsing the Michael Line in Avebury, following its energy patterns as it travelled in a south-easterly direction between the row of magnificent standing stones, known as the West Kennet Avenue, heading for the Sanctuary (originally a stone complex and part of the sacred Avebury landscape). As I was dowsing outside the Avenue, and I found a series of three 'energy lines' that were very different to the energy patterns of the Michael Line.

I found them on the other side of the line too, they seemed to be holding the power and vitality of Michael between them. I called them 'Shepherd Lines' as they seem to guide Michael from one sacred site to another. I wrote to Hamish, asking if he had found the same lines, as they hadn't been mentioned in *The Sun and Serpent*. He replied that he had and called them 'Outriggers'. He was delighted that someone else had also found them, and I was so pleased that Hamish had been able to verify what I had discovered.

These outriggers, or shepherd lines, help contain and direct the power of these wonderful energy channels. As they run through the sacred sites you can only imagine the patterns and memories from the past and present, they have absorbed on their journeys.

Living above or on one of these lines can be detrimental to your health, partly due to the human emotion contained within them, also the earth energy patterns that they have picked along their journey, interacting with all the sacred sites.

Don't forget that not all people and animals are affected the same way.

118

You may start to feel off colour whilst others may find the energies exhilarating and invigorating, everyone reacts differently.

When I am dowsing for a client, I like to map the energy channels exactly as they run though their home. Most lines, such as a spirit lines or fault lines will have a gentle shape to them but are, in the main, straight and I draw them on the plan as such.

However, energy channels twist and turn, so they need to be mapped correctly.

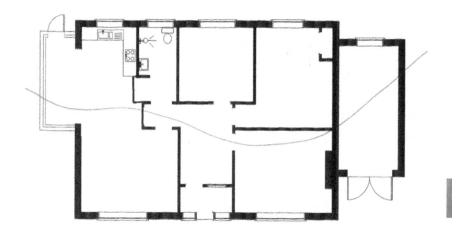

*Energy channels on a floorplan*

Start by finding out where the energy channel enters the house (let's say it does so from the left hand side) and mark this location (I often use a pencil so that I can rub the marks out later), move your pointer an inch or so to the right and start moving up from the bottom of the plan until your rod or pendulum moves (do this slowly so that it gives your instrument time to move) and again mark the location. Keep doing this until you have reached the other side of the house, take out a light blue pen and join up the dots. You have just tracked an energy channel.

You may find that you have two or more energy channels affecting your home, do check how many you have. Crossing points are referred to as nodes. Hamish and Paul found many as they followed and dowsed the

Michael Line (energy channel). It wasn't until they arrived in Avebury that they discovered a second line, now known as the Mary Line (energy channel). They eventually realised that the node points were, in fact, where the two lines actually crossed. They then had to retrace their steps back to their starting point in Cornwall eventually plotting the Mary Line and her interaction with Michael.

## Case Study: Dinner with Michael

After teaching the first day of my *Heal Your Home* course in Glastonbury, I was invited for supper at a friend's house. Little did I know what was in store. I walked up the High Street, past St. Michael's church, turned left at the T junction and their home was a short distance along the road.

I was greeted with a cold beer, just what I needed after talking all day, and we sat in their living room discussing the course, general dowsing, healing, Glastonbury and the Michael and Mary Lines. After about half an hour I started to feel rather strange, floaty and ungrounded, and then came a feeling of vertigo. Was the beer really that strong? I looked over at my hosts and they both seemed to have a wry smile on their faces, or was that my imagination?

I excused myself and headed for the cloakroom, purely to sit down in peace and quiet and sort myself out. I carried out a grounding exercise, dowsed to see if I needed to clear any energy patterns that might have attached to me during the day, but there were none. So, I boosted my psychic protection, which is very much needed if you are visiting the Glastonbury area.

After a few minutes I started to feel slightly better. I walked out of the cloakroom and dinner was being served so we adjourned to the dining room, and as I sat down the same odd feeling began to return but this time it was much weaker, it seemed boosting my protection was helping. The wry smile was still there, and I was just about to ask what was going on, when it dawned on me, I was sitting directly on the Michael Line and had been in their living room too.

They saw the understanding on my face and said 'Welcome to dinner on the Michael Line, we wondered how long it would take for you to realise. Certainly, much quicker than most people we have had here in the past.

Interesting isn't it?'. Not the word I would have necessarily used, but yes, it was an experience.

Once I knew what was causing the feelings, it was easy to tune in and harmonise myself to Michael's energy patterns, it became a warm fuzzy feeling in the background, rather like wrapping a blanket around yourself. But the intensity that I was initially exposed to could easily have been debilitating had I not had my protection on already. I was not sure how the couple survived living there, but as I have said before, there are those lucky people in the world who are bullet proof, and nothing affects them. Me, I have to work at it.

As I left the house, I thanked them both for a very interesting and entertaining evening, and as I walked back down the High Street to the George and Pilgrim Hotel I sent as much light and love as I could to the Michael energy channel, I needed to as it ran underneath where I was sleeping that night as well.

## Case Study: Annie

We went out for a walk one day, with Annie, our springer spaniel, parking the car on a side road in Ripon. Allyson and I got out and donned our walking boots whilst Annie sat very impatiently in the boot waiting for us to finish.

10

The walk took us along a beck (meaning a small stream in Yorkshire), and we joined the Ripon Rowel, which is a 50-mile circular walk around the Ripon countryside, that eventually leads to Fountains Abbey and its extensive grounds. All was well with Annie until we arrived at St Mary's church and the grade II listed obelisk (circa 1805) next door to it. She was not happy and did not want to go near either building.

Allyson was keen to see inside the church, leaving me and Annie outside. I went to sit on the obelisk, but Annie was determined not to go anywhere near it, which was very strange behaviour for her. So, I picked her up and carried her over, placing her on the wide ledge and sat beside her. She kept looking for Allyson, and her gaze was fixated on the church door. I got my mobile phone out and walked a short distance away and took her photograph, she just sat there, immovable and staring, also rare behaviour for Annie.

In the photograph, that we looked at later, she looks disconsolate and vulnerable. She relaxed slightly when she saw Allyson coming out of the church, but it wasn't until we were at least 100 yards away that her tail started wagging again. As you move away from the church you look down a long dead straight road that leads directly to Ripon Cathedral, a ley for sure, and of course, you will have the energy channels feeding into it.

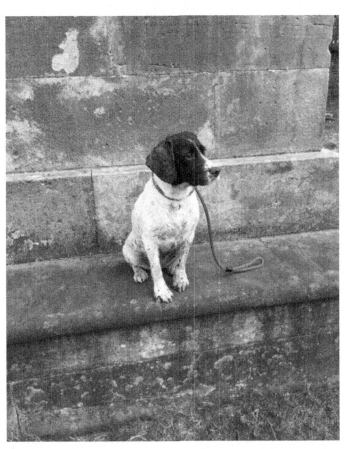

*Picture of Annie looking very pensive*

Later on, I printed a close scale map of the area and started to plot the lines, finding that a powerful ley runs directly from Ripon cathedral, through the church and obelisk. There were also two energy channels meeting and crossing at the obelisk. It is a very energetic place and worth visiting if you are ever in North Yorkshire. But perhaps not with the dog.

Annie didn't like the energy patterns at all so, on our next visit, Annie and I stayed well back and admired the view from afar.

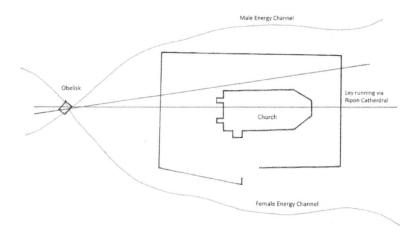

*St Mary's Church and Obelisk, Studley Royal, Nr Ripon, North Yorkshire*

## Dowsing diagnostic questions for energy channels:

1. Is the home or family detrimentally affected by an energy channel?
2. If so, how many?
3. How detrimental are they on a scale of 0 to -10?
4. Is there a crossing point in the house?
5. Does the line or lines contain any detrimental human emotion?
6. Does the line or lines contain any detrimental earth energies?
7. Once cleared, will there be any more layers to clean and harmonise?
8. Are there any spirits associated with the line?
9. Is it beneficial for them to be helped into the light?
10. If so, when is the best time to do it?
11. Can it/they be diverted away from the home and other that the affect detrimentally?
12. Am I allowed to do any further healing of the energy channel?

# 11. Fault Lines

I have always known about fault lines in the earth, they are commonly found in tectonic plate collision zones, and have created mountain ranges like the Rockies in the USA, the Alps in Europe and the Himalayas. The most famous, or should I say infamous, is the San Andreas fault line in California. The plates are constantly moving and as they do, they create these imperfections in the earth. Some are massive, like the Rift Valley in Africa, whilst others are so small, they cannot easily be detected by the human eye, but can be found through dowsing.

## Case Study: Belas Knap

Despite my knowledge of fault lines, what I had not realised, was the close association between fault lines and sacred or holy sites. It was not until I heard Alan Neal, a well-known and respected west country dowser and author of *'Dowsing in Devon and Cornwall'*, giving a talk on the energies found at sacred sites that I started to take notice and then, once I had delved deeper, I decided that I needed to include them in my questions relating to geopathic stress and people's homes.

During his talk to the Earth Energies Group, Alan mentioned that almost every sacred or holy site that he had visited and dowsed had one or more fault lines running either through it or very close to it.

We were due to visit Belas Knap the next day, an ancient Long Barrow on Cleve Hill close to Cheltenham and Winchcombe in Wiltshire, so I made a note to myself to dowse the site once we got there. The evening before our visit, I had a vision, a mental picture, looking down on the site from above and saw the fault line running close to, but not through the long barrow.

The next day was sunny, as it always seemed to be on the Earth Energies Group weekends, and we all met in Winchcombe before walking up hill to the site. Although the Long Barrow has been restored over the years it is still an energetic site and worth visiting. As with any dowsing group meetings, once we got there everyone scattered, all doing their own thing. Some were chanting in the entrance to the barrow, some looking for pictograms on the ground, others were dowsing energy lines and leys. Me, I went to look for the fault line.

I asked my rods to show me where the fault line ran, and they pointed to the eastern boundary, so I walked until they crossed, I had found it. The line ran diagonally across the site from the northwest to south east, but it did not run directly through the long barrow. That would have been madness on the part of the builders as the long barrow would not have survived for long with the constant movement along the fault, and they would have likely been aware of the existence of the line when they were building.

The line was extremely lively, and you could feel what I can only describe as a slight crackle of energy beneath your feet. I asked if the people who constructed Belas Knap knew that the fault line was there and got a Yes.

I started to ask questions to find out more about the relationship the fault line had to the site:

*Does it factor in the overall energy of the site? Yes.*

*Does it contain similar patterns to earth energy lines? The rods wavered, so on to the next question for further clarification.*

*Does a fault line contain earth energies as well as human emotion? Yes*

I needed to find out how it differed.

*Do fault lines vibrate at a similar level to a bog standard (if there is such a thing) earth energy line? No.*

Now we are getting somewhere.

*Are they energised all the time? No.*

*Do they need regular human interaction to power them up, at sacred sites? Yes*

This next two questions were the best.

*Do we physically need to be on site to keep the energy flowing? No.*
*Can we do this purely through thought? Yes.*

So, by just thinking about a site, wherever you may be in the world, you can energise it. Isn't that amazing?

## Case Study: Guernsey

Several years later, I was teaching an Earth Healing course in Guernsey, and we had set up a small stone circle in a local hall the day before and left it overnight to see what energy patterns it would attract. We had dowsed the best location for its construction, the number of stones needed and where they should be placed.

I admit that I had not given any thought as to whether there was a fault line there or not.

The next morning, we gathered in the hall. Nigel Clarke who runs Queux Plant Centre on the Island walked into the circle and was almost thrown out by the guardian spirit. Seemingly he had not entered respectfully and therefore paid the price. He hadn't thought to check if there was a guardian there, an error any one of us could have made, and ask its permission to enter the circle. We were all very careful after that, the circle was now considered a sacred site with its very own guardian attached.

We did some dowsing during the morning and found that an energy channel had diverted itself and now ran, temporarily through the centre of the circle, energising it, also an energy spiral had appeared, which hadn't been there the night before. It certainly made the meditation interesting and everyone seemed to get something from it. One or two connected with the guardian, whilst others went on a spiritual journey.

After the tea break, I suddenly got the compunction to dowse for a fault line and found one connected, energetically, to the circle. No one had noticed what I was doing so I asked if anyone wanted dowse to see if we

126

had a fault line in the hall. Several did and found it almost exactly where I had a few minutes earlier. It was just outside the circle, rather like Belas Knap, close enough to influence what we were doing but far enough away to not to interfere with its stability.

One of the attendees asked, 'Would there be visible signs of a fault line?' Good question. I suggested that we go outside and have a look at the wall, it had been rendered and painted white some time ago, making any damage easy to spot. As we approached the area that we had pinpointed a few minutes earlier inside the hall, we saw there were cracks running up the wall at the exact location.

We were all delighted, not just for finding the fault line, but also that we had placed the stone circle so close to it and had been able to harness its energy.

Although a fault line helps sacred sites 'power up', it is not good for humans and animals to permanently live within its energies. It would be detrimental to most people, certainly in the long term. In the short term? Remember that some people do not get affected by geopathic stress, but it is always best to check that your home and family are clear, just in case you are all sensitive to the harmful energetic effects.

With the plan in front of you, ask whether the house and any member of the family is affected by a fault line, if yes, then you need to locate it on the plan. Run your pointer or finger along one wall, asking to be shown where the fault line is, if there is no movement then run your pointer along another wall and see if the rod/pendulum indicates the presence of the line. Once it moves mark the spot with a pencil, then you could either ask the rod or pendulum to show you the direction the fault line runs or move the pointer to a different wall and ask to be shown its exit point.

Mark the location and join up the dots, I tend to use a light green pen.

When mapping fault lines on a house plan, I tend to draw them in as a straight line but, in reality, the line is likely to deviate slightly. You will not go far wrong by plotting it as shown on the plan below and then, by asking the right questions, find out how far to either side and above the detrimental effects can be felt.

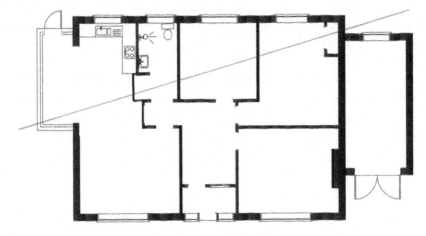

*Fault Line on a floorplan*

## Dowsing diagnostic questions for fault lines:

1. Is the home or family detrimentally affected by a fault line?

2. If so, how many?

3. How detrimental are they?

4. Can they be healed and harmonised?

5. How much of the energy within the lines is inappropriate human emotion?

6. Can this be cleared?

7. How much of it is earth energy linked?

8. Can this be cleared?

9. How long is the line (as a matter of interest)?

10. Will it remain clear or are there layers to be worked on?

# 12. Dynamic Energy Lines

As we know, there are many different types of energy lines surrounding the Earth, and it is useful to be able to categorise them. By identifying and naming them, and the energies flowing within them, helps us with the healing process, and it is showing respect to Mother Earth and all her complexities.

I had been mystified for some time that whenever I went into a cave system (which is not that often) and dowsed, I could never find any, what I would term, earth energy lines. Hamish had mentioned finding or dowsing a form of energy lines underground in one of the books he had written, but when I asked the question 'Are there any earth energy lines here?' I got no reaction from my rod or my pendulum, which is my 'no' response.

Either Hamish was wrong, or I was, but I would have placed a bet on it being me. Then I started thinking, was I asking the wrong question, being too specific or not specific enough? I dowsed and got yes; I was. I needed to find another way of querying and quantifying what Hamish had found as I was sure there was something there.

I remembered attending a weekend course with Hamish and Ba, and during the first day he was dowsing for a 'hot spot' in the room. This is an area where various energy lines coordinated and once found, you then started to focus all your thoughts on this location. As you did so it expanded and produced more radials or spokes, it reacted to human consciousness, and often produced a spiral and a lemniscate (the Infinity symbol).

Hamish would ask 'How many radials were there at 4 o'clock this morning before anyone came into the hall?' The answer may have been eight or less, but he had established a baseline to work with, and that is what I needed to do while I was in a cave. I knew then that I was being too specific with my questioning so, the next time I was underground, I was determined to set my baseline and hopefully find this elusive energy line, or whatever it may turn out to be, I was not going to be fussy.

Ingleborough caves were about an hour's drive away, so off I set with my collapsible dowsing rods in my jacket pocket. It was quite a walk from the car park to the cave entrance and when I arrived there was a group of seven people gathered, including the guide, ready to descend into the cave.

As we got further into the cave, I held back a little, assembled one of my rods and formulated my baseline question. 'Are there any energy lines down here as described by Hamish Miller?' I went straight for the jugular, no messing around. The rod gave me a yes response. 'Are they earth energy lines as I would view them?' No.

I had found out what the problem was, I was asking the wrong question, better still, I was asking the right question but the wrong way. I was being too rigid, or specific, in my phrasing. I asked the rod to show me where one of these lines were and found it about two feet away. I followed where it pointed and stopped when the rod moved, indicating that I had found the outer edge. I was overjoyed, I had finally solved the mystery of Hamish's missing energy lines, but what to call them?

I couldn't just label them as an 'earth energy line' as they contained a different type of energy to those I had already detailed in my house healing report and I needed to differentiate between them. It was not until I was working on *Spirit & Earth* with Tim that the word 'dynamic' suddenly came into my mind.

And so, Hamish's lines are now referred to as dynamic energy lines.

They are similar to earth energy lines, in that they both run along the surface of the earth; however, the energetic output of dynamic energy lines will also be found many hundreds of feet below ground level. These dynamic lines, like a 'normal' earth energy line, can also interact with human consciousness, expanding and contracting in width.

This human interaction was no more apparent than when I taught a course in the Avebury Community Hall. The energies in the hall changed, subtly to begin with, as the attendees chose their seats and readied themselves for the day. Earlier I had dowsed to see if the hall contained one of these dynamic lines and it did. I then went about measuring its width before anyone entered the hall, and found it to be around 2ft, then, just before I started talking, I measured it once again, to find it was slowly expanding. Then an hour later I dowsed again to find that it had increased in size, now encompassing all the attendees in the room.

We all drew upon these increased energies during the course; however, I would not want to live in that heightened state permanently. It would not have just been the information contained in the course work that could cause the attendees fatigue, the dynamic line would also be the culprit.

Living within these expanded and higher vibrating energy patterns 24/7 would certainly be very harmful to many humans, therefore the lines need to be cleared and healed of any harmful energy patterns running within them, which includes a percentage of detrimental human emotion as well as earth energy problems.

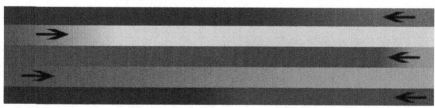

*Energy bands flowing in opposing directions*

Unlike earth energy lines, dynamic lines are made up of varying numbers of energy bands, each band travelling in opposing directions. I never seem to find even numbers of bands, only odd, like 3, 5, and 7. I usually check how many of the bands need clearing and then carry out healing on each one. As these lines interact with humans, it is therefore logical to assume that like water veins, they can absorb and store our emotions.

People go to sacred sites for many different reasons, some to dowse, some to soak in the ancient energies, and some to let go of their stress and worry. By just sitting or walking around somewhere like Avebury, relaxing and unwinding, much pent-up emotion can be released.

## What do you think happens to it?

If every sacred site becomes an emotional dumping ground, and those emotions are never cleared away, can you imagine how the sites would feel when you visit? Sinister is one word, depressing is another. They would become places that no one in their right mind would want to go to for any length of time. So, there must be a way of keeping them clear, one that doesn't have to involve human beings, and dynamic lines play a big part of this, allowing detrimental patterns to flow out of the site, dispersing and diluting them over many miles as they wend their way across and under the countryside.

Imagine what living above an active line could be like?

## Case Study: Disturbed Sleep

In August this year, Allyson and Annie were not sleeping very well. First, I checked to see the current cycle of the moon, but it wasn't close to full or new, so that wasn't the cause. Because I now mostly dowse using my eyes (an upward movement for yes and a downward movement for no) I started asking question, from my checklist in my mind.

*Is it a lost soul? No.*

*Is it problems with a water vein? No.*

*Is it earth energy related? Yes.*

I then worked through the various lines connected to earth energies, including vortices or energy spirals. I narrowed it down to a dynamic line and found that several of the individual bands contained energies that were detrimental to Allyson. I then questioned why and found out that it was to do with the energy around Covid-19. The emotional outpouring of hundreds of people had infected four of the seven energy bands. Their fear, anxiety and uncertainty was pouring out of their homes, infecting the dynamic line, which then ran through our home.

No wonder both Allyson and Annie were having problems, however I seemed to be okay. I set about working on clearing the bands and sending the appropriate healing to those people who were responsible for infecting the line in the first place. I wanted to see if what I had found and the healing work that I had carried out would make any difference to their sleep patterns before I told Allyson what I had done.

The placebo effect is of course a factor in any healing, and if Allyson had known that I had been working what was disturbing her sleep, then if there was a change, it could be put down to that. So, I did not say anything and waited to see what would happen. The next morning, Allyson came up to me and said, 'Have you been working on me?' I asked why. 'I slept really well last night, first time in about a week'. I then explained what I had found.

Locating them on your plan is the same process as fault lines, and they again tend to be reasonably straight as they run through your home but may have a slight curve. I normally use a purple pen to mark them.

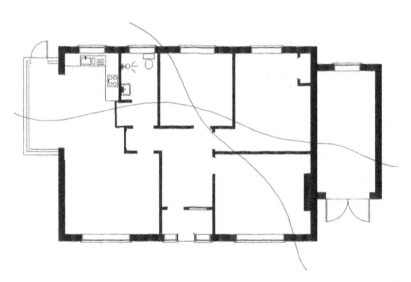

*Dynamic energy lines on a floorplan*

## Dowsing diagnostic questions for dynamic energy lines:

1. Is the house or family affected by a dynamic energy line?

2. If so, how many?

3. How detrimental is each one?

4. How many bands are there running in each dynamic line?

5. How many of them have been affected by the detrimental energy?

6. How far above and to either side can the detrimental effects be felt?

7. Can healing be given to them all?

8. If no, when the next healing can take place?

9. Can the whole line be cleared?

10. Am I allowed to divert them from the home and others that they affect?

11. Can I send healing to all the other people who live on or over the lines?

12

# 13. Human Intent Lines

For those of you who have read *Heal Your Home* or have attended any of my talks or courses, you will recognise a change in the name. Originally, I referred to human intent lines as leys or holy lines, due to their connection with sacred sites like Thornborough Henges in North Yorkshire, Arbor Low in Derbyshire or Long Meg and her Daughters in Cumbria.

All the above sites have at least one thing in common, they will have a line running through them, sometimes several, and many of them are connected by these remarkable lines. They are found in churches, cathedrals, and abbeys, just as much as stone circles, henges and burial mounds.

Why the slight change in the name? Well, I believe that many, if not all of these lines have been created though human intent. Yes, there is undoubtedly a holiness to them, however I now look at them as an energetic guide or pathway leading from one sacred site to another. Now this goes a little against Alfred Watkins original description of a ley line which was, '*a straight alignment drawn between various historic structures and prominent landmarks.*'

But I do feel, in his defence, that if we as modern-day humans look at an odd, shaped rock, hill or promontory and go wow, what must our ancestors have imagined. Was it made by some strange being or a God? It could easily have become a venerated site, then being linked, by human intent, to another such site, just down the road or many miles away. An energetic network of human intent lines connecting up all the ancient sacred sites, not just in the British Isles but also around the world.

My first book contains a lot more information on these fascinating and dowsable lines. Finding them on a plan is again quite straight forward, follow the guidelines detailed in the fault lines chapter. I usually marked them in brown when drawing up the plan.

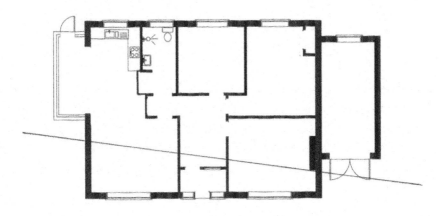

*Human intent line on the floorplan*

## Dowsing diagnostic questions for human intent lines:

1. Is there a human intent line running through the home?
2. How many?
3. Where are they?
4. Are they detrimental to the family?
5. How long are they?
6. How many sacred or notable sites do they cross or join?
7. Does healing need to be sent to each site?
8. Can the complete line be healed?
9. Is there a layer system in place? (If so, when can I heal the next layer?).

# 14. Energy Spirals

Energy spirals or vortices are created by the crossing of two or more lines, whether water veins, energy lines, stress lines and so on. Neither of those lines need to contain any detrimental energy for them to form a spiral that is harmful to you and the family. And on the flip side of the coin, if two or more detrimental lines cross in your home, they create a vortex, but that may not be harmful, it may be neutral or even beneficial.

The energy spirals should not generally be moved or interfered with, as the energies from them are needed to help bring balance. However, they do need to be harmonized, enabling us to co-exist with them, and ensuring that life continues on this planet due to the free flow of energy. If this wasn't case then we would, perhaps, see a blockage occurring and the pressure would begin to build. The sudden released of this pent-up energy could produce a spike or surge that may upset the equilibrium of the planet.

14

It's a good idea to find out as much as you can about the spirals and vortexes, whether they are spinning upwards or downwards, clockwise or anti-clockwise, whether they are masculine or feminine in energy, and how far from the centre the detrimental effect can be felt.

Once you have cleared and harmonised the detrimental energies from the spiral, they can be good places in which to work. But a word of caution as the energy patterns can still be a little intense, especially after sitting above and in a vortex for long periods of time.

They can also be good places for meditation but do check to see which spiral is the best for you that day. You may have a number rising through your home and each one will have a different energy. Sometimes you may need to sit in a masculine spiral, whilst on another day a feminine one would be more beneficial, because our DNA is made up of both x and y chromosomes. I have often found that anti-clockwise spirals are more detrimental than clockwise spirals but check to see if that is the same for you.

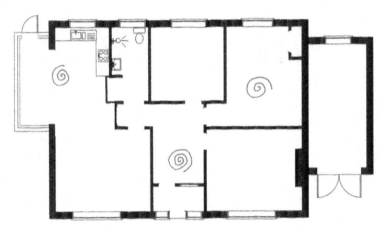

*Energy spirals marked on the floorplan*

## Dowsing diagnostic questions for energy spirals:

1. Are there any detrimental spirals affecting the house?
2. How many?
3. Where are they?
4. How detrimental are they?
5. Which direction do they rotate?
6. Are they spinning upwards or downwards?
7. Do they have a masculine or feminine energy?
8. How far either side are the detrimental effects felt?
9. Can I harmonize all the detrimental spirals?
10. Is there a spiral that is beneficial for me to sit on?

# 15. Energetic Sink Holes

There is a slight change in the title I used in *Heal Your Home*, with the addition of the word 'Energetic', as I find that this is a more accurate description.

They are small naturally occurring holes that allow energy to flow from one dimension (ours) to another. They are not harmful by nature, but when situated in your home, especially in a well-used area, they can become very detrimental to your health.

If you are standing above, or close to, one of these energetic sink holes, they can drain your life force – that is, from the auric field that surrounds you.

Unlike the family that I wrote about in *Heal Your Home*, it is extremely rare to find one in your shower cubicle, I have certainly never found one like that since. But they could be situated under your bed, favourite chair and so on. It is worth checking for them as they can be very draining, and over a long period of time, debilitating.

15

## Case Study: Lucy the black Labrador:

As part of my house healing, I often get asked to dowse the family pet, to make sure that they are healthy, have no elementals attached or bothering them and that they are not being affected by any detrimental energies.

Along came Lucy, the love of the family, and by all accounts a beautiful happy and bouncy dog when outside, but became timid, had a lack of energy and was very restless in the house. 'It was just like switching a light off,' said the owner. 'No sooner does she walk through the back door and go to her bed; the life seems to go out of her'.

They had sent me a plan of the house, but I had asked them not to mark where Lucy's bed was situated. I like to work quietly through my questions and see what I find, rather than being shown where a problem area might be. They had a utility room and larger kitchen/breakfast room, but I felt that Lucy's bed was not in either of those rooms, I felt that her bed was under the stairs in a large alcove.

This proved to be the case, and directly under her bed was an energetic sink hole. The poor little lass, every time she went into her bed, her life force was constantly being drained. It was being sucked from her, so it was no wonder she didn't have any energy.

I carried out a healing on the location straight away, even before informing the owners what I had found. I wanted to make sure that Lucy did not suffer any longer. I made sure that the detrimental aspects were cleared, and the sink hole sealed. I also sent healing to Lucy to speed up her recovery.

I called the owners to bring them up to speed, and I just managed to say hello before an excited voice said 'Have you been working on Lucy? She is so much better, her tail is wagging, she greeted us when we came downstairs and suddenly seems full of beans, we have Lucy back.' That is exactly what all of us involved in healing love and need to hear. Especially when a pet reacts that way, as Lucy obviously did not know that the healing was taking place, therefore there was no placebo, just the pure channelling of energy from the Universe.

The family were delighted, and they asked if they should move Lucy's bed, but I said no, that it was now her special place, harmonised and safe.

When showing the location of an energetic sink hole on a plan I tend to use a circled black *

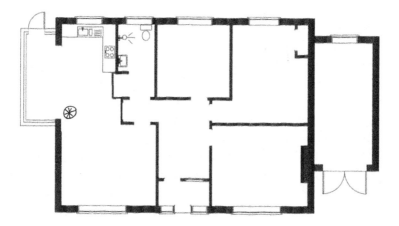

*An energetic sink hole marked on the floorplan*

## Dowsing diagnostic questions for energetic sink holes:

1. Are there any sink holes in the house?

2. How many?

3. Where are they?

4. How detrimental are they to me and the family?

5. Can they be sealed for all time?

6. Do I need to do anything before sealing the sink hole?

7. Will I, or the family, start to feel better once the hole is sealed?

15

# 16. Reversal Points

These are naturally occurring phenomena that have come up a few times in past investigations. I am finding them less and less though as the years go by and it does feel that they are closing themselves down without the need for human intervention. They are simply energetic places that allow the energy of the planet to rise freely into the atmosphere, but when covered by an object, say a bed or a table, the flow is blocked. The rising energies have to find themselves another exit point and when they do it tends to be very detrimental to humans and animals.

A reversal point is an area that, if kept clear, is harmless, it allows the energy patterns to flow naturally. The actual reversal point may be situated outside, but if obstructed in any way it can allow/cause noxious energies to permeate and rise in your house.

If one is found you can either keep it uncovered, or as I found out during a house healing, you can also seal them.

It is worth checking every few months just to make sure that your home is not affected by a reversal point as they can be very harmful to the family if covered.

I tend to mark a reversal point with a red asterisk on the floorplan.

16

## Dowsing diagnostic questions for reversal points:

1.  Are there any reversal points affecting the home?

2.  How many?

3.  Are they inside or outside the house?

4.  Where are they exactly?

5.  How detrimental are they?

6.  Can I seal them?

7.  Do I need to clear the house of their detrimental effect first?

8.  Will they remain sealed for all time (If no, then check to see when you need to carry out the next healing session)?

16

# 17. Emotional Energy Areas (Human Conflict)

Emotional energy areas are exactly what they sound like. They are areas that have been formed as a result of highly charged emotional situations. They can occur in both your home and workplace, and once created, will often be the trigger point for further emotional situations, as they grow in intensity.

Humans are emotional beings. Love, passion, hate, jealousy, and envy are all emotional responses to external stimulus. They dictate how we react to certain situations that we find ourselves in, either helping, due to a calm emotional state, to get ourselves out of trouble or perhaps by being hot headed digging ourselves into a deeper hole.

We need emotion, we need the passion it brings out in us, but we do need to ensure that the output of any outbursts does not energetically build up and become detrimental to our health and wellbeing.

We all vibrate at different levels at different times, and we can leave these traces of ourselves behind, especially when we move to a new house, and these energy patterns could turn out to be very detrimental to the new family. I firmly believe that is why the 'Divorce House' syndrome exists, a property that repeatedly comes onto the market every three or so years due to regular family break ups.

Though you can, of course, win an argument, everyone would lose out in the aftermath, especially if the detrimental energy created by the

17

dispute is not cleared. So, if you find yourself in an emotionally charged situation, once things have calmed down, dowse to see if any emotional energy areas have been created. If they have, and in all likelihood, they probably will have been, use the exercise detailed in healing section to quickly diffuse and clear them.

If you remember to do this, perhaps even on a daily basis, you will find that the argument trigger points will lessen over time as you will not be influenced by the build-up of any detrimental energies from past conflicts that could have easily intensified and begin to press your buttons.

It's important not to forget to clear the other person involved in the argument, as they may have been influenced by detrimental attachments. You may suddenly find that they come up to you and give you a big hug, or offer an apology, after the healing has taken place.

Be sure to check for any detrimental energetic bed patterns as well. We leave emotional traces on our beds when we get up in the morning, both good and bad, depending on our dreams and state of mind when we went to bed.

It is better to leave the bed in a neutral state or you may find those bad dreams you had the night before, returning.

## Dowsing diagnostic questions for emotional energy areas:

1.  Does the home have any emotional energy areas?
2.  How many?
3.  Where are they?
4.  How detrimental are they?
5.  Are they inherited?
6.  What caused them?
7.  When were they caused?
8.  Can they be healed?
9.  Will there be another layer to heal later on?
10. Do I need to find a way to stop them happening?
11. Are there detrimental bed patterns?
12. Can I clear them today?

17

# 18. Psychic Cords

Psychic Cords are thin silver threads connecting one person to another. They are normally linked to our chakras and they become attached for many different reasons, some good and some not so good.

Affection is a major factor in psychic cords being created, and will link one lover to another, heart chakra to heart chakra. A mother sending healing thoughts to a member of the family who is ill can also subconsciously link her heart chakra to their solar plexus chakra, transferring her life force energy across to assist with the healing. Our subconscious minds are capable of this.

The problems happen after the couple part company, leaving the cords attached, or when the family member has made a full recovery, but the mother's energy is still flowing out. Gradually, all those involved will feel the ill effects.

All parties are bonded together until they are consciously freed, or the cords cut, and this can be debilitating over time. In the case of lovers, it can create the feeling that neither of them is able to move on with their lives, especially if one person does not want to. The attached cord can be used by one person to control consciously or sometimes subconsciously their ex-partner. In the mother's case, she might feel tired, listless, and unsettled, finding sleep difficult as she would still be psychically linked to the member of her family, as well as physically and mentally.

18

So, it is therefore worth checking yourself weekly or monthly for any detrimental psychic cords that might have attached to you, check your family regularly too.

The healing section describes how you can easily cut these conscious and subconscious cords, but a word of caution. If you find a cord and then sever it do be aware that the person who attached it, or it was connected to, may suddenly feel that something has happened, or feel that an energetic change has taken place. They may not understand but the chances are that subconsciously they will, resulting in you receiving a text, email or telephone call from them, out of the blue.

If that happens, you will need to check to make sure that they have not attached another psychic cord to you. Follow the same procedure, cut the cords, checking both front and back of your chakras. Psychic cords can appear like an octopus, tentacles all over the place, so it may take a little bit longer to disentangle and cut them all the first time, but it should get easier after that.

## Dowsing diagnostic questions for psychic cords:

1. Do I have a psychic cord attached?
2. How many?
3. Who attached the cord, me or the other party?
4. Who is the cord attached to? (i.e. parent, child or friend)
5. When were the cords attached?
6. Where are they attached? (i.e. to the physical body, aura or chakras, don't forget to ask whether at the front, back or both)
7. Can they be cut? (if yes, then do so, if no, ask when you can do this days, weeks or months)
8. Is there a good time in which to do this?
9. Will this be beneficial to me?
10. Will this be beneficial to the other party?

18

# 19. Dimensional Portals

Since writing about fourth-dimensional portals in *Heal Your Home*, I have become aware that there are many more dimensions than four, so we need to check for portals to these other dimensions when we are dowsing our home. We also need to be aware that we naturally open doorways or portals as we carry out our dowsing and healing work. These need to be firmly closed once we finish our work.

As with most healing modalities, when we channel energies from the Universe, certain chakras open to receive this healing energy and in doing so a dimensional doorway or portal is created. This allows the free flow of divine light into our body, via our solar plexus chakra, this is then sent out to those whose names come into our conscious and subconscious minds.

They can also be opened by repetitive detrimental thoughts, depression, playing with a Ouija board, computer games (as we have read about in the sorcery/black magic chapter), illness and so on.

If you have found an open portal or doorway in your home, it will need to be closed as soon as possible.

'Spiritual Hygiene' is so important here to prevent these from staying open. When I finish my healing sessions and dowsing work, I make sure that I close myself down (see healing section), clearing away any energy patterns that may be detrimental and ask that any doorways that have been open expectedly or unexpectedly during my work are firmly closed and that any residue that may be left behind is removed and taken to the light.

Some of the doorways you come across may well have been opened for years, so before you close them make sure that all and any beings that may have come through are sent back to their own dimensions first, and then ask the Archangels to help you clear away any residue or detrimental energies that they have left behind.

## Dowsing diagnostic questions for dimensional portals:

1. Is there an open dimensional portal in the house?

2. Where is it?

3. How long has it been open?

4. Have I opened the doorway during any of my healing sessions?

5. Have any of my family been responsible for opening it?

6. Is it detrimental to me and the family?

7. How detrimental is it? (0 to -10)

8. How was it opened (i.e. depression, stress, on purpose, healing session, computer game)?

9. Can it be closed?

10. Can I do this today?

11. Should I clear away any detrimental energies that may have come through the portal first?

12. Once closed are there any further energies that need clearing?

# 20. Illness Trigger Points

This new concept came to me several years after I published *Heal Your Home*, because of tragic circumstances. It relates to an exact point in time when you, both mentally and physically, have reached the end of your tether and that memory becomes trapped in your cells. It can then, potentially, rear its ugly head once again, at a later stage in your life when you find yourself under pressure.

It is often said that stress, worry, angst, or trauma held in the body has to come out, and it can appear as a rash, constant headaches or migraines, hair falling out or changing colour (that is how mine manifested itself during my business years) and various forms of minor illnesses.

It can be released through healing, therapies or a change of lifestyle, but if you keep it bottled up inside and do not deal with it, then it could be years later when it finally manifests, and by then it is more difficult to heal and release.

## Case Study: Hidden Trauma

For some time, I had been working on a client and her family. She was a wonderful strong lady and we had built up a strong rapport over that time. She had previously been diagnosed with cancer of the stomach, had been through chemotherapy and when I began working with her, she was in remission.

When she called me, she explained that she wanted the house healing carried out for her family so that she knew they were safe after she passed away. She had always felt that the house had a strange energy to it and that it may have been the cause of her illness.

I explained that when I worked on a home, the whole family were also a major part of the healing process, because everything and everyone would need to be brought into balance and harmony. I began the process and once completed, I sent the detailed report and drawn-up plan, explaining and showing where the problem areas were in the house. There were several water veins and various energy lines that ran very close to where she slept, and they may have been the catalyst to her illness.

She had explained in her initial call to me that both her parents had died of cancer and it had always worried her that her family had a predilection for the disease. After the initial healing, we had a number of follow up telephone calls, because feedback is so important to me when carrying out any form of healing. She reported that the family dynamics had changed for the better, her teenage children seemed happier, her husband less stressed, and in her own mind she felt much better and more relaxed.

As with many of my clients, we became friends, and we spoke regularly over the next few years. Then in one of those calls she said that the cancer had come back. She had been for a recent test and the doctors had confirmed it.

The first words out of my mouth were 'What happened to you when you were 14 years old?' The words just came into my head and I felt I had to say them. She went silent for a moment and then said, 'I can't talk now as we have friends over, can I call you back once they have gone?'

She called back a few days later. 'What did you mean when you asked me what happened when I was 14 years old?' I explained that I had heard the words in my head and had to repeat them. She then went on to explain what had occurred:

'When I was 14, I was raped by my uncle. Both my parents were out, and he and I were alone in the house. It only happened once as I made sure that I was never put in that position again. I didn't tell my parents as I felt both embarrassed and guilty, perhaps I had led him along and somehow it was my fault what happened.

'I found myself pregnant and went to the local doctor and explained to him what had happened, I asked that he not tell my parents or call the local authorities. He was incredibly understanding and organised for me to visit a local clinic to terminate my early and unwanted pregnancy. If I had kept the child, my parents would have needed to be told the circumstances and I could not let that happen.

'My visit to the clinic went by in a haze, I remember little about it. I went home and continued with life as best I could. They say that time heals all, but I could never rid myself of the guilt I felt. Was it my fault, did I do something to encourage my uncle? Why me? Had I done something bad and needed to be punished?

'So, Adrian, apart from me, my doctor and the lady that performed the operation, you are the only other person that knows about what happened to me when I was 14 years old. I have never even told my husband.

'That puts you in a very small minority. I admit that I never thought that I would ever tell another living soul about what happened. Then along you came. I admit that I have bottled it up for years and I suddenly feel so much better finally being able to tell someone and get it off my chest.'

I kept very quiet as her tragic story unfolded, and all I could do was send healing thoughts to both the grown woman and the young girl still stuck inside her. Guilt, abuse (mental, physical and spiritual), shame, shock, and violation were all words revolving around my head.

I could not, and still cannot, imagine how that 14-year-old girl must have felt, and how she found the inner strength to do what she did, all by herself. What a brave young girl she was. We now needed to do a lot of work on the inner child, to find a way to clear her of the guilt she felt and allow her to move on, to enjoy the rest of her life.

I asked that she give me a couple of days to sit down and work out a healing programme. I freely admit that I sat for a long time afterwards trying to gather my thoughts. I realised that I had been put into a very privileged position, not just by the message from Spirit, but also by being trusted with her story, now I just needed to figure out what to do next.

I sat quietly and tuned into what I had been told, and the words 'Illness Trigger Point' came flooding into my head. It was then that I knew what to do. All healing takes place at a cellular level, but I needed to go back in time to when the attack took place and start the healing process at a cellular level from there.

That is when, I felt, that her cells started going rogue. The shock to both her mind and body caused them to mutate and then hide, and this started the process that eventually morphed into cancer. It was understandable but felt sinister.

I'd always felt that the healing I carried out would go deep enough, but it just shows that sometimes you need to dig even deeper, to ask specific questions, to get the answers and then carry out the necessary healing in whatever form it takes.

It all sounds very logical to me now, but at the time it was something new. I find that the Universe will always keep testing me, and constantly throw new problems my way. I then have to work on finding the solution to them. That way, they keep me moving forwards, and as the energy patterns of the earth change, I do too.

The conclusion to the story was that with healing and her newfound happiness, we managed to keep the cancer at bay for another three years. She and her family decided to forego any further chemotherapy as it made her feel so ill, so she stopped all her prescribed allopathic medicine and just lived her life.

We spoke many times over that period, and she said that she felt so much calmer and at peace, able to accept, in her own mind, that she had not been the guilty party. 'I feel free for the first time since the attack happened,' she told me.

That was the last time we spoke.

We had booked in a time to talk but no call came. I waited a few days, as I know life can get busy and I was sure she would ring me at some stage during the week. The call never came, so I rang her number, and a man answered the telephone. I asked to speak to her. 'Sorry' he said, 'she passed away peacefully last Wednesday'. That was the day we were scheduled to speak.

20 I admit to shedding a few tears that day, for such a lovely lady and who was so strong right up until the end of her life on this planet.

I still think of her.

Since that day, I have delved deeper into illness trigger points to find out how they affect us and why they are caused. There can be many reasons, not always as dark as in the story above. Stress, anxiety, childhood diseases, teenage angst, death of a loved one, relationship break ups, the worry and pressure of exams/achieving good grades, jealousy, bitterness, hatred, trauma, can all be part or the whole cause of a later illness.

## Dowsing diagnostic questions for illness trigger points:

1.   Does my body/mind suffer from an illness trigger point (detrimental cellular memory)?
2.   When did it happen (what age and date)?
3.   Can this be put down to an illness or accident?
4.   If not, was it due to a different form of stress (bad relationship, memories, anxiety, etc.)
5.   Is there any other cause or trigger point?
6.   Is this something that can be worked on to clear it?
7.   What work is needed (forgiveness of others or self)?
8.   Is spiritual healing the best way to deal with it?
9.   Would therapy help to clear the memory?
10. Has this cellular memory been passed on to offspring? (this is very rare)
11. Is there anything else I need to know?

# 21. Consecrated Ground

None of us really know what has occurred on the ground which our home is built upon. We might know what has happened in the short-term perhaps, but not what was there, say, a thousand years ago, or even several hundred. There are maps that may give us a clue, but unless you dowse the question, you may never know.

Most people would consider consecrated ground to be a churchyard or where other religious buildings stand. And though this is true, consecrated ground does not have to be Christian or religious in origin or even related to physical buildings. Our Pagan ancestors worshipped from temporary altars; the whole of Mother Earth was sacred. Giant oak trees, for example, were seen as a conduit between the heavens and earth.

Ancient stone circles, henges, standing stones, long barrows and sites like Brimham Rocks in North Yorkshire and many of the White Horses (possibly Dragons) in Wiltshire could all be described as consecrated or sacred. Should they be demolished or ploughed in, as many were during the First and Second World Wars, their energy patterns would still be in existence, the ground still considered holy and therefore need to be deconsecrated.

Deconsecrated means to transfer (a building or site) from sacred to secular use.

As an estate agent (in my former life) we often came up against an ancient

'Chancel Repair Liability' or 'Church Tithe' on our vendors deeds. A shock to both them and the buyer. It meant that the local (or sometimes not so local) church can legally require you, as the owners of former rectorial (church) land, to meet the cost of their repairs, and this can be backdated for many years.

I have come across whole villages whose homes are built on what is still considered as sacred or holy land. Several housing developments, including much of Woodbridge Hill in Guildford, had houses sold on 99-year leases, the church being the freeholders. (This was in the 80s and 90s, it might have changed now).

So, by implication, is your home then built on consecrated land? If the church owns or has owned it in the past, does it make it the land holy?

Yes, it does. But why should this matter?

Everything on this planet vibrates at different levels, including the land, buildings and, of course, people. It is good to visit a sacred or holy site, as the energies found there can be quite exhilarating. But if you stay too long, they can become draining. You certainly would not want to live on or within a sacred site on a permanent basis.

Because consecrated land is probably vibrating at a higher level than is safe for us in the long term, it is a good idea to find out, through dowsing, if your home has been built on holy ground. You may live in a converted church or chapel and find out that it hasn't actually deconsecrated, this can easily be rectified by following the healing exercise in Part Four.

Though they would not be considered holy, any buildings that have had their original use changed, will also need to be cleared of their old energetic patterns and the new use established, especially if converted to residential. We cannot call an old mill, for instance, sacred or holy, but if it is converted into apartments, as many have been, it's best for the new residents to ensure that all the old energy patterns are changed accordingly. It is, if you like, a form of reprogramming.

## Case study: Converted School

This was the case for a former school building that I worked on. The couple had purchased an old village school as it had closed due to the lack of pupils attending, and it was no longer a viable option to keep open. They had spent a lot of money tastefully refurbishing it, but they told me it had never really felt like home.

The reason?

Energetically it was still a school, and no one had told the building otherwise. Even though the classrooms were now converted into beautifully decorated living accommodation, the bricks and mortar still held the essence of education, the original use of the building.

So, in essence, I had to approach the 'planning authority' Upstairs to ask that all the old energetic patterns left behind by the pupils and staff were removed. I cleared any mental and physical abuse that had been created by both the teachers and students, also anxiety, emotional upset, stress and fear as well as four spirits that needed help to go to the light.

The footprint of the building also needed work as the original room layouts had been changed with walls being removed to make the accommodation more user friendly. The energetic imprints of the old walls needed to be erased, wiping the slate clean. Subconsciously, the original walls and doorways were still in place and stopping the free flow of energy around the new layout, leaving each room energetically stymied.

It works the same for any house extensions and loft conversions, you will need to clear away all the old energetic footprints that existed, and incorporate the new build into the existing house, for it to actually become one complete home.

## Dowsing diagnostic questions for consecrated ground:

1. Is the home built on consecrated ground?
2. Has the house been used for prayer meetings or gatherings in the past?
3. Has the land on which the home is built been used for sacred gatherings or ceremonies?
4. How far does this date back (AD or BC)?
5. How long was it used for?

6. Was it a temporary altar place?

7. Was there a sacred site or building here in the past?

8. Was it a Church, Chapel, Meeting House, Pagan hut?

9. Does it affect me and the family living in the home?

10. Therefore, is it detrimental to me or a member of the family?

11. (If you live in a converted chapel or church) Has it been deconsecrated?

12. Can I de-consecrate the area/ground today?

13. Are there any spirits connected to the site that need help?

14. Are there any old wall or door imprints that need clearing away?

15. Are all the rooms fully incorporated, energetically, within the house?

# 22. Curses and Spells

A spell does not necessarily have to be cast with intent, or with magical ingredients and specific wording, but it does need a certain amount of emotion behind it to make it work.

Random thoughts are therefore very unlikely to have a detrimental effect, but strong, repetitive emotions or thoughts directed at a person or a place, along with a verbalised wish, will, almost certainly, produce a spell that will not dissipate until it is discovered and lifted. A curse, however, is something much deeper, darker and deliberate.

Jealousy, envy, and hatred are some of the main reasons why curses come into existence. If someone has hurt you or your family in the past, repeated deep emotion and detrimental thoughts directed towards them, can easily create a curse. The opposite can also be true, and you may find a curse directed towards you, so be on the lookout for this. Finding out the reason why is important, as it will help you get it lifted.

Never fight fire with fire, as it only makes things worse. It is all about forgiveness (or understanding) and unconditional love. Why did the person curse you or send a spell? Why did you send a curse or put a spell on them? All of this will have come from either your conscious or subconscious mind, theirs too.

None of us are innocent, we have all been in difficult situations in the past, been dealt with or spoken to harshly, or dealt out hurtful words ourselves, so we need to ascertain that there are no spells or curses cast by us that are still current, as well as making sure that there are none working against us.

Animals, particularly horses, can also be the recipient of a curse or spell. I have come across several cases in recent years, most have been through jealousy. Jealousy of a friend who thinks her horse has a better connection with another rider or that someone else's horse is preforming better than their own. The horse too can get jealous.

A lot of spells and curses have been placed on land rather than people, especially where planning permission has been submitted and the neighbours have vehemently fought against it. This can create a lot of animosity, especially if successful.

Repetitive dark thoughts or lingering upset can easily conjure up a spell or curse, and this can affect the land and house for years, causing problems for the poor unfortunate family buying the house 30 or 40 years after it has been built.

You will find that in many cases, the curse will have been set in the distant past, the person who cast it has passed over many years beforehand. It is a good idea to make sure that the person responsible has actually gone to the light as this makes the problem easier to solve, mainly because there is no longer a reason for the spell or curse to remain.

When carrying out the healing it is always good to send light and unconditional love to the person that cast the spell or curse as well as the recipient.

## Dowsing diagnostic questions for curses and spells:

1.  Am I or the family affected by a curse or spell?
2.  Is the house affected by a curse or spell?
3.  Is the land affected by a curse or spell?
4.  If it is a spell, how many?
5.  If it is a curse, how many?
6.  How detrimental is it/are they to me/the family?

7. Were they/was it cast on purpose?

8. Was it a subconscious thought?

9. How long has it been in existence?

10. Is the person that cast it/them still living?

11. Can the spell/curse be lifted?

12. Can I send healing to the person responsible?

13. Are there any spells or curses still current that I have been responsible for?

14. Can I lift them and send healing?

15. Are any of my pets/animals the subject of a spell or curse?

16. Is so, can they be lifted by me?

17. If not by me, who can do this?

18. Is there are reason why (jealousy, your dog might have bitten or snarled at someone etc.)?

19. Have any members of my family been responsible for sending a curse or spell?

20. Is so, who and why?

21. Can these also be lifted?

# 23. Psychic Attack

We are living in a time of extreme comparison. It is perhaps natural to feel envious or jealous of someone who has more than you, or who has the relationship/job/car/home you want. But it is these extreme feelings of resentment and jealousy that can cause a psychic attack on those people that have what you perceive you want.

Despite the saying that anger and bad feelings can only hurt you, psychic attacks can be instantly detrimental to the person who is being targeted. You, or someone you know, may be sending harmful thoughts for a multitude of reasons. Unlike curses and spells, that are almost always conscious thoughts and physical practice, psychic attack will, more often than not, come from the subconscious mind.

Work-related psychic attacks are one of the most common, the person who felt that they should have got promotion instead of you, jealous of your relationship with fellow workers, even down to your dress sense. Psychic attacks regularly occur in relationships too, an ex-girlfriend or boyfriend (wife/husband) not happy with you or the breakup, or jealous that you have successfully moved on and are happy with a new partner.

The detrimental thoughts, by themselves, are not necessarily going to cause someone harm, but when they are charged with a lot of emotion, repetitive and sustained for long periods, they begin to have a damaging effect.

The effects of being psychically attacked can include insomnia, headaches, anxiety, bad dreams or night terrors, joint pains, heart murmurs (if the attack is constant), brain fog, an inability to concentrate and feeling unsettled.

## Celebrity Attacks:

Psychic attacks can increase the more you find yourself in the public eye. So, if you are well-known in any area, for any reason, you really do need to protect yourself.

I have worked with some well-known celebrities, several of whom have said that they felt elated when they landed a part, but within a few days there had been a backlash, almost a wave of depression that overtook them, and one or two complained of the sudden onset of a headache.

I found that some of the many hopefuls, who also auditioned for the same part, were subconsciously attacking the successful actor, because of their extreme disappointment and dissatisfaction in not landing the part. The detrimental thought patterns, feelings and deep emotions had been directed at the successful candidate who was chosen for the part, causing them to suffer the onset headaches and a mild feeling of depression.

I presume that footballers may probably feel the same animosity directed at them by the opposing teams' fans, and the same would apply to many team and individual sports.

We all need to protect ourselves, more so if you are in the limelight, as there is a lot of jealousy out in the world and unhappy or discontented people often feel the need to have someone to aim at.

We are all capable of sending as well as receiving these detrimental thoughts, so as well as making sure that you are not affected by a psychic attack from someone else, it's also good to make sure that you are not guilty of doing the same, either now or in the past.

If you are guilty of creating any psychic attacks in the past you will need to make sure that you have cleared these harmful energies and thought patterns, sending the affected person healing and a spiritual apology. And do remember to forgive yourself, so that no detrimental energy of guilt remains.

By working through the questions, you should have a good idea who, if anyone, is sending the detrimental thoughts yours or your family's way, and why. It's often due to jealousy and envy, but the reasons can go much deeper and darker. Also, to find out whether it is on purpose or a subconscious reaction.

## Dowsing diagnostic questions for psychic attack:

1. Am I under psychic attack?
2. How detrimental is it to me or the family?
3. Can I prevent it from happening?
4. Do I know the person involved?
5. Is it a family member?
6. Is it a friend?
7. Is it a work colleague?
8. What age are they?
9. What colour hair do they have (natural or dyed)?
10. What is the motivation for the psychic attack? (Money, envy, etc.)
11. Have I been under psychic attack in the past?
12. When did this happen?
13. Who was responsible? Use questions 4 – 8.
14. Can I carry out a healing?
15. Can I send healing to the person responsible?
16. Will sending healing stop the person from attacking me in the future?
17. Have I psychically attacked anyone in the past?
18. Can I send them healing now?
19. Will it be beneficial to them?
20. Will it be beneficial to me?

# 24. Power Artefacts

My first career, straight from school, was in antiques. The company that I worked for in Mayfair, London, specialised in late 17th and early 18th century oak and walnut furniture, which to me, were the most beautiful materials and an amazing period for craftsmanship. I often used to wonder what kind of life a particular oak refectory table had gone through, who had sat around it, what did they talk about, had it gone through good and/or bad times, and what memories did it retain?

That was a long time before I had even begun to think about any forms of healing, but there I was, wondering about the life a table had led, and what emotions may have sunk into its very fabric. Even then, at times I felt that certain items of furniture had a warm glow about them whilst others felt cold, almost neglected.

Many years later I have found myself clearing those very same items of all unwanted and detrimental energy, most of it from deep human emotion. Any object is capable of attracting detrimental energy which can then affect people within its proximity.

## Case Study: A painting hanging in a house in the West Country.

I was contacted by a lady who had attended one of my *Heal Your Home* courses. She had missed out on the second course, hence the call. She had recently moved to a new house, could not settle and was feeling rather uncomfortable, almost as though she wasn't welcome. I was asked to carry out a full healing on it, to rid the house of any old energy patterns left by previous owners.

This I duly did, working through all the questions, producing a detailed report and drawn-up floorplan. During my investigative work, I found a power artefact in her living room, I cannot remember how detrimental it was but there were some quite nasty vibes being given off.

When carrying out this work I don't ask for or get sent any internal photographs, so I never have an inkling of what the infected article might be when I find one, or more, in a client's house. It might be an item of furniture, ornament, piece of jewellery or an artefact that they have brought back from a trip abroad. It can be time consuming, but I like to have a go at identifying the offending article.

In this case it was a large painting hanging in a prominent location within the house and when I saw it in my mind's eye, it appeared as swirls of blue in many different hues, no discernible picture, just a mass of blue. I picked up that it was the artist who had caused the painting to become detrimental, it was full of their frustration and dissatisfaction of the finished article. I carried out a clearing and healing to make sure the painting was balanced and peaceful in its surroundings.

What I did not realise is that my client was a well-known artist and that she had painted the power artefact herself. We did have a chuckle about it afterwards and she admitted that, in her own mind, she could never get the colours right. It was supposed to represent the blue of the sky, melding with the blue of the sea. 'I over painted it several times,' she said 'and felt that I could never get the colours quite right. Yes, I was frustrated but perhaps exasperated would a better word to use. All I wanted to do was throw it into the sea and be done with it. I persisted but was never satisfied. My father loves it, hence the reason for it hanging in my house, I am still not sure though.'

I do feel that clearing away the energetic patterns that had soaked into the painting helped, and I believe that it is still hanging in her home, in pride of place, and hasn't caused issues since.

I know that she will laugh when she reads this.

*Update:* In early 2021, I was approached by my client to check her house as she'd had some building work carried out. Generally, the house was fine, there were a few emotional energy areas to clear and some minor earth energies and two water veins, but what I did discover is that the painting was still being badly treated. It came in at -2 in detrimental effect, much less than before but was still the object of the artist's ire. It has been cleared again and this time has a protective bubble placed around it.

## Case Study: Unidentified object in Norfolk

Sometimes it is very difficult to determine what a power artefact is, even if you get a vague picture in your mind. This was the case when I was working on a client's house in Norfolk.

I picked up on the energy of the object in question in my client's living room and all that I received as a picture was mangled metal. I admit to wondering why anyone would have twisted metal in their home. I had heard of people having their old cars crushed and placing them in their large hallway as a focal point, but this was not a big room and my client did not seem the type to have done this.

The questions went roughly as follows:

*Does it stand on the floor? Yes.*

*Does it have feet? Yes.*

*Is it a table? No.*

*Could it be used as a table? Yes.*

*Confused? Yes* (that was how I was feeling)

*How high is it, can I count in feet? Yes, it was roughly 3ft in height.*

*What is it made of? I ran through various materials and found out that it was cast iron.*

So, we had a piece of mangled cast iron that could be used as a table, but it wasn't a table. I gave up and literally wrote that in my report and sent the whole thing off to my client.

I received a telephone call a couple of days later, as I like to run through the report and try to answer any questions that my clients may have on the information supplied. I was also interested to hear about what the mangled metal object actually was.

We ran through a lot of the questions until we got to the mystery object, 'You were so close' she said. 'Yes, it does indeed look like mangled metal, but it is the base of an old Singer sewing machine, probably from one of the factories that were around here. I bought it and had a glass top made for it so that it can be used as a side table'.

The detrimental energy came from the women that had toiled over it, working long hours for very little money, fatigue, fear of redundancy and so on. What we would now call a sweat shop, but in the early days was the norm.

The table was cleared of all its detrimental energies, from the past and present, leaving it in harmony with the house and owner.

## Case study: Spaghetti Tin

I was dowsing a lady's home and came across a power artefact in her kitchen. You can imagine the thoughts going through my head had she committed a crime using a sharp knife, hit someone over the head with a meat tenderiser, or hurt herself in an accident?

Thankfully it was none of the above. It turned out that she had just gone through a particularly nasty divorce and had literally started her life afresh. New home, all new furniture, all new crockery and cutlery, there was nothing left over from her marriage, except a spaghetti tin.

It had been given to them as a wedding present from special friends and it was the only thing that she had kept, not for the memories, but for the bright colours and size. And it was the only power artefact in the whole of her new house.

I had identified what it was and where to find it in the house, and she was both impressed and also aghast that the one object she had kept was infused with detrimental energy from her failed marriage. That really was the key as to why it was so detrimental. Many of their arguments had taken place in the kitchen and for some obscure reason the spaghetti tin had absorbed much of the detrimental energies given off.

168

After I carried out a healing on the tin, I assured her that it was now clear of any old emotional patterns, so she did not need to throw it out. She was thankful as she said it would have been impossible to replace.

## Dowsing diagnostic questions for power artefacts:

1. Are there any power artefacts in the house?
2. How many?
3. Where are they?
4. Why did they become detrimentally charged?
5. When did they become detrimentally charged?
6. How detrimental are these power artefacts to the family?
7. Can they be healed?

If you are working remotely, and you cannot just walk around you home to find them you can ask these further questions:

8. What is the item made from? (Wood, metal, porcelain)
9. Does it stand on the floor?
10. Is it an item of furniture?
11. Is it an antique or modern (20th or 21st century)?
12. Table, chair, stool, bed, cabinet, sideboard?
13. Does it hang on the wall?
14. If it does, is it an oil painting, print, tapestry?
15. Is it made from a precious metal?
16. Is it a ring, watch, pendant, brooch, earrings, pen?
17. Could it be considered a family heirloom?

24

# 25. Place Memory

These areas are darker and more detrimental than the emotional energy areas you find in most houses. They are mainly caused by the continued deep human suffering and physical injury that have marred the place, it can last for decades or even centuries.

Battlefields, both ancient and those from more modern times, will contain many of these areas, created by bloodshed, agony, fear and anguish from both humans and animals alike. If you take a trip to Verdun on the France/Germany border and walk through the surrounding forests, you will get a sense of exactly what a place memory feels like, especially at the French Forts at Douaumont and de Vaux.

Vimy Ridge, in the Nord-Pas-de-Calais region of France, is another. Try walking around the surviving trench system. They have been restored, but there is still a feeling of death and destruction in the air, even though a lot of healing work has been done there, especially by Allyson and myself.

Our own homes can also be affected by these energies from the past. Just like consecrated ground, we don't know what might have occurred beneath the settee where we like to sit and watch television. Your study or healing room may have had someone buried beneath it hundreds of years ago (I have found this several times), their remains have completely disintegrated, but the energy of their passing still exists and can be very detrimental to you and the family, including your pets. The energy patterns will need to be worked on and healing sent.

If a place memory problem is found when dowsing a floorplan, I tend to start with what date the problem occurred, and then find out why the detrimental energy still remains as there may be an underlying cause and understanding what it is will certainly help the healing process. Look for any discarnate souls that might be connected to the place memory as they will need to be dealt with before you carry out any further healing to the area.

## Dowsing diagnostic questions for place memory:

1. Is there a detrimental place memory within the home?
2. How many?
3. Are there any in the grounds of the house?
4. Where are they?
5. How detrimental are they?
6. When do they date from, AD or BC?
7. What century?
8. Why did they occur?
9. Can they be healed?
10. Are there any lost souls who need to be moved on before healing the place memory?
11. Will there be any others to move through later on?
12. If yes, then when?
13. Are there various layers to heal?
14. Any subconscious layers to heal?
15. Do I now need to do some healing on the earth itself, to rid it of any detrimental energy patterns left by the place memory?

25

# 26. Interdimensional Place Memory

These are obviously similar to place memory (25) but with a twist. The best way for me to explain what they are, is tell you how I found these extraordinary energy patterns in the first place.

## Case Study: Smells from an Unknown Source

It was several years back, and I was working on an innocent-looking bungalow in Lancashire, which turned out to be nothing of the sort. It was, what I would call, a 'learning property', as a lot of what I found there was new to me and was subsequently added to my checklist. The lady who lived there was very gifted, although she felt it was more of a curse, because she could see spirits and elementals (nature spirit) amongst other things.

My client told me that she regularly saw a spirit sitting on her neighbour's doorstep. It seemed to be a local portal, and extremely popular one at that. She then went on to describe how she frequently, both saw and heard, the joyous singing of elementals along her own garden hedge.

During the clearing and home healing I performed, I helped close to 100 spirits move through to the light.

It was during this time that both she and her husband mentioned to me about a curious smell in their study that was beginning to permeate into their hallway. When I asked what it smelt like I was told manure, but not manure, perhaps more like silage (the preserved green foliage crops that is fed to cattle and/or sheep during the winter), it was sweet and acrid.

The first thing that I checked on was whether it was a lost soul or a life/ thought form, but no, it was neither of those. I thought then that I had better ask the very open question 'Have I dealt with anything like this before'? The rod partially moved, meaning that I had worked on something similar but not exactly the same.

The questions had to continue:

*Has this smell been there all the time? No.*

*Has it been there before? Yes*

*Was it before I started working on the bungalow? Yes.*

*Are we talking about weeks or months? Months.*

*So, is it seasonal? Yes.*

*Was it there the same time last year? Yes.*

*The obvious question came next:*

*Is it the smell of silage? Yes.*

I called them and asked whether they lived next door to a field of cows, they replied not anymore there are houses all around us and have been for many years. That was not the answer then.

More head scratching went on, but I was determined to find out why the smell was there.

I asked the owners if they knew whether there had ever been a barn there before the bungalow was built, but they did not know. It had obviously been a field at some stage, but the bungalow was built sometime in the 50s. More than enough time for any country smells to have dissipated.

Back to the drawing board. I ran my eyes down my checklist and they seemed to stop on 'Dimensional Portals', ah ha, my eureka moment.

*Is it a dimensional portal? No.*

*What do you mean, no?* I was getting exasperated.

*Okay, is it like a dimensional portal? The rod slightly moved – I was on the right track, again.*

26

*Are we looking at a past or present memory coming through? The rod twitched again; I was getting closer.*

*Could I call it a place memory as it does not affect the whole of the bungalow? Twitch of the rod.*

*Is it from another dimension (in desperation)? Yes.*

*So, should it be thought of as an interdimensional place memory? Yes.*

I had finally got there. The smell was coming from another dimension, a place where a barn existed, built in exactly the same location as the bungalow in this dimension. As the cows were brought in for the winter, they would start to eat the silage, and that was the smell affecting my clients.

Really? My first thought was, could this be true?

I decided to carry out a healing before I told the couple what I had found, just in case they thought I had lost it, big time.

As I tuned in it felt like a tear in time, or perhaps a better way of describing it is, a thinning of the veil between us and the different dimension. This then allowed the detrimental energy, or smell in this case, from a parallel Universe (dimension, hence the new title) to flow through and affect my clients in their home.

A week after I had worked on this problem, I got a call saying that the smell had completely disappeared, and they asked what I had found and what had I done. I told them about the parallel world and how I had found out and then carried out the healing.

Their comment was simply 'Oh right, well done'. They were not phased at all. Since then, there has been a lot of talk about multiverses, perhaps this is what I stumbled across, unwittingly.

Though I have only found a few since, it is worth checking for, as the veils do seem to be thinning between worlds, and more so at different times of year.

The more people talk about these other dimensions the more they can become ingrained in our psyche. It is therefore important that any healing we carry out includes these other dimensions or universes, just in case. We have yet to fully comprehend how our actions in this world affects those people living in other dimensions, therefore an awareness is needed when working on any form of healing, to include as many people as we can, in any universe.

## Dowsing diagnostic questions for interdimensional place memory:

1. Is the home affected by an interdimensional place memory?
2. If so, when does this date from?
3. What has caused it to happen?
4. Are there any spirits attached that will need moving to the light?
5. Human, animal, or both?
6. Will there be any other layers to heal?
7. Can they be done at the same time?
8. If they cannot, can I put a date into my diary?
9. Can the tear or thinning veil be repaired after the problems have been traced and dealt with?
10. Will this heal the problems that have been experienced?

26

# 27. Vows or Contracts

One of the biggest vows that we can make, which you could also call a contract, is the vow of marriage. You are not only making this vow in the eyes of the law, but also in the eyes of God. It doesn't matter where the wedding took place, whether in a church, chapel or mosque, a boutique wedding or on a beach in Hawaii, (and it doesn't matter what your religion) here on Earth, God or the higher power, has the final say.

You say, 'I do', or a form thereof, exchange rings, jump over the sticks, sign the Marriage Certificate, have a party in the evening and then off you go on your honeymoon. But have you ever thought about where the words, 'I do' actually go after you have said them? I admit until I started working on vows and contracts a few years back, I didn't think about it either.

I received a vision when working on a client and her vow, it came from the beginning of a film called Contact starring Jodie Foster (1997) that has the most amazing opening scene (You can be view it on YouTube if you are curious) which had the answer. It starts off focussing on a city with a close up of some buildings, then begins to slowly move upwards, away from the earth. You start by hearing people talking, modern music playing, car horns blaring, public speaking and this continues as the 'camera' moves through space at an ever-increasing rate, past the moon and then the planets, finally leaving our Solar System.

The chatter remains in the foreground, and as it moves further away from

Earth, the older the music becomes, and you hear part of Churchill's 'On the beaches' speech. It keeps going and going, beyond known space, but still the noise is there, travelling forever through the dark void.

It has been scientifically proven that light travels in waves, and that the light from a star twinkling in the night sky has taken thousands, if not millions, of years to reach Earth. Sound works the same way, so all the noise we humans generate does not just stop when it reaches the person sitting in front of us or at the end of our cell phone. Our words may end up travelling past our known Universe into the beyond for ever.

It's an intriguing thought that someone out there could be listening to your solemn vows, even though they were made many years ago.

Divorce is a natural part of life these days, there are of course still couples who have been married for decades, some even celebrating their landmark Ruby Wedding Anniversary (40 years). But there are many who won't get to that magical moment, me included (I haven't got enough years left to do so). Split marriages are so common that it is rare to find children still living with both their biological parents.

So, we return to the marriage vows. The breakup has happened, you obtain the Decree Nisi and then wait until the Decree Absolute arrives to finally nullify the marriage. A great day for some, not so good for others.

In the eyes of the law, you are no longer a couple, but what about the vow to your God of 'Till death do us part'? Those words are still out there, in the ether. They need to be rescinded, with all spiritual links to be cut. This allows you both to go your own ways in peace, without a forgotten and invisible knot still tying you together. There may also be some psychic cords still attached, but those should have been discovered in section 18. It's always worth checking again though.

Vows come from inside you and are made live by your conscious thoughts and then they sink into your subconscious. Therefore, they impact on your very soul, which is what makes you, *you*. You will need to ensure that you have not made any other vows throughout this life and to check whether they are still current, and you still wish to uphold them.

As well as vows of marriage, there are vows of chastity, silence, faith, poverty, surrender to God, stability, fidelity, obedience, humility, peace, and so on. Though you may not have made such vows in this life, it is believed that these vows can follow you from a previous incarnation and affect you in this one.

In recent years, I have also found that you can be affected by a simultaneous life vow as well. There are parallel versions of you, living lives in different dimensions alongside this one. And the vows that they make could affect you, and you making and breaking of vows in this life could also adversely affect them. In section 30 I go into more detail about these other lives and dimensions and how they affect us.

The following example shows the effect a vow can have on our lives. The names have been changed.

## Case Study: Sisters in Cheshire

I was first approached by the eldest sister, Sophie, to carry out a healing on her new home. She had recently moved in and wanted to clear the house of the last owners' energies. There had been an acrimonious divorce, and she did not want to be affected by anything they may have left behind them.

This was duly carried out and the house was given a 'spiritual spring clean'. About nine months later, I received a telephone call asking if I could help her sister Joanne who was in a spot of bother. She sent me all her details including full name and date of birth, plus her address, actually two addresses, as she had recently moved back to her parents' house because she was badly anorexic and needed to be looked after.

My first port of call is always to check whether a spirit was linked to her and to clear any nasty attachments that might have taken hold. There were no spirits, but I do remember that she had a number of attachments at -7 in detrimental effect. She lightened up considerably after that, but there was something else lurking and I just needed to work out what it was.

The background to her returning to her parents was a sad one. Through hard work, she had earned a place in a renowned University and after spending her first year in the Halls of Residence, her parents decided to

27

buy a flat for her to live in. They had found a modern apartment close to where she was studying, bought new furnishing, gave her a helping hand to move in, and all was well.

That was until Sophie went to visit her several months later, and as she walked in she was shocked to see that there was no furniture left in the apartment, the cooker and hob had gone as had the washing machine, microwave oven, and most of the cutlery. Her sister was sleeping on the floor in a sleeping bag as there were no beds either.

'Have you been burgled?' asked Sophie.

Joanne had a confused look on her face. 'No, why do you say that?'

'The flat has been devastated, everything has gone including most of the kitchen, what happened?'

'I gave it all away', said Joanne 'I didn't need any of it'.

'My sister had always been a little scatty and her head was always in the clouds, we just put it down to the fact she was intellectual and saw things differently to us,' Sophie explained to me. 'But this had gone far beyond anything she had done in the past. She had lost a lot of weight and was a shadow of her former self, I was worried, not just for her physical health but also mental.'

Sophie called their parents and told them that she was bringing Joanne home, that she needed help and to arrange a doctor's appointment. It was put down to depression and pills were prescribed, but after several weeks she still had not put any weight on and that is when Sophie decided to call me.

'Can you have a look at Joanne and see if you can find anything that might have accounted for her giving away everything in the flat and her reluctance to eat, please?'

Of course, I agreed. I started with the apartment and did not find anything there that would have accounted for her strange behaviour, but I still carried out a healing and left it clear of any past detrimental energy patterns. Then I did the same for her parents' property, to make sure that she had not taken anything nasty home with her, making sure all was clear.

I then started working on Joanne. Yes, the attachments were quite detrimental, but there was little there to explain her bizarre behaviour. I asked Upstairs if I was missing something and got that I was.

*Have I come across anything like this before? No, was the response.*

*Does the problem stem from her current life? No. It could have been from bullying at school, a feeling of inadequacy, lack of confidence, sibling rivalry, exam stress and so on. But it was none of those.*

*Is it to do with one of her past lives? Yes. (I had not yet started looking at parallel lives.)*

*Is it a curse, spell, vow, contract or something similar? Yes.*

*Is there more than one? Yes. It is always worth asking this extra question.*

So, I had narrowed it down to two vows from a past life that were responsible. I just needed to work out which ones. There was a vow of poverty, that was logical, the other was a vow to God, and she had become a Nun.

In that life she had abandoned all belongings, avoided any attachments (worldly goods, friends and family) and finally, after a number of years, decided to devote her life to God and the church. No wonder then that she found living in her new home difficult. As she spent more and more time by herself, she must have begun to experience echoes from her past, gradually these took over and she finally had to get rid all the luxuries surrounding her.

For Joanne to make a full recovery I had to find a way for her to release these past memories, allowing her to lead a normal life today. This was achieved partly by me invoking her guides and higher self and also Joanne having to verbally rescind any past and present contracts or vows.

It took time for her recover. She gradually put on weight and her parents stopped worrying. She quickly came off the anti-depressants and started to talk about a return to University to finish off her studies. I lost touch after that but did say that if the family ever felt she was going backwards to contact me. I have not heard anything, so I assume that all is well.

Contracts are very similar as they can be made in this life or come from a simultaneous or parallel life. They often involve family members or close friends; however, business partners can also form part of a contract. They can often be debilitating, and feel like you are being controlled, emotionally drained and may eventually lead to a physical and mental burn out.

When I first wrote *Heal Your Home*, I was still looking at karma and how, if we made a mistake in a past life, it could lead to us having to repay the debt in this life, but I am beginning to view things slightly differently, as my thoughts turn once again to parallel lives (Section 30).

I originally viewed vows or contracts as karmic debts, but because they have such an impact on our lives today, I feel that we now need to view them in other ways. As we have seen with interdimensional place memory, energies from other dimensions are leaking through to our own, this can mean that any vows made in one of your simultaneous or parallel lives can have a major effect on you in this current existence.

Do not forget that vows are linked to individuals, you spoke the words therefore you need to make sure that the vow is fully rescinded. 27

## *Dowsing diagnostic questions for vows or contracts:*

1.  Do I or does any member of the family have a vow or contract that needs lifting?
2.  Is it from a simultaneous life?
3.  Is it from this life?
4.  Is it from a past/parallel/simultaneous life?
5.  Was I, or the member of the family male or female at that time?
6.  What date does the vow or contract come from?
7.  What type of vow or contract was it?
8.  Why is it still in existence? (Lesson to learn etc.)
9.  Can it be lifted?
10. Can it be done today?
11. If not today, when can the work be done?
12. Can I lift or remove it?

13. Does the person also need to be involved in the lifting process?

14. Are there any cords to be cut during the lifting process?

15. Is there another person that needs to be involved or informed?

# 28. Fractured/Torn Souls

When dealing with fractured souls over the last few years, I have often found that a tear described the problem better rather than referring to it as a fracture or break, hence the slight change in the title. (In *Heal Your Home*, I called this section 'fractured souls'.)

Sometimes you will find a tear in one's soul from the moment they are born, especially in the case of an unplanned pregnancy, an unwanted child or one who is going to be put up for adoption. I do believe that we are aware of our surroundings very soon after the female egg has been fertilised, so parents need to be aware of this fact and try to be very careful what they say and/or do throughout the pregnancy, otherwise their actions and words can have an adverse effect on the unborn child.

With the world population growing exponentially, it is logical to assume that there will be many more babies being born with torn or fractured souls; I have certainly found this to be the case. If the tear is small, they will grow up slightly unsynchronised, a part of them damaged until a healing occurs.

When I find these soul tears in children, I have often been told by the mother that her pregnancy wasn't easy, or that there were psychological problems in the relationship, or that the father had abandoned them part way through, and possibly mental/physical abuse had occurred.

These tears can diminish our natural psychic protection, which is the auric field surrounding our physical body. I feel that the soul is to be found in the 4th layer (Astral) and the 5th layer (Etheric Template) of our aura, and if any part of it is damaged, even with one small single tear, it can allow external detrimental energies to enter and/or attach to us, further adding to the child or later on the adult's problems.

Therefore, we need to repair the damage before we can do anything further to help. The Archangels are always there to help us carry out this repair work, they are spiritual tailors armed with a holy needle and thread.

I would view a fractured soul the same way, the problems that caused it to split are very similar to those detailed above. To me there is very little difference, if any, and I am purely using terms that you may be more comfortable with, or have read about before, in my first *Heal Your Home* book for instance. I feel that the terms can be interchanged depending on your viewpoint. The main thing is to find out if there is a problem and then do something about it.

## 28 *Dowsing diagnostic questions for fractured/torn souls:*

1. Do I or any family members have a torn or fractured soul?
2. Which member is it? (Unless you are very specific this can include your parents, in laws, aunts and uncles, or grandparents)?
3. How bad is the tear/fracture in percentage terms?
4. When did this happen? (Do not forget to include before birth)
5. Why did this tear or fracture happen?
6. Am I able to repair or heal it?
7. Can I use an Archangel to heal?
8. Does any part of the soul need to be retrieved?
9. Once the healing has taken place, do I need to put further protection around the soul?
10. How long will this protection be needed?

# 29. Stress/Disturbance Lines (Man-made)

I have yet to find a home that does not have one or more of these lines running through it. Depending on what caused them in the first place will determine how detrimental they are to you and the family. Some people will have a severe reaction to them whilst others are shielded by their body's own natural defence mechanism, a strong auric field.

As the title suggests, these lines are the result of human interference on the planet, earth disturbance is one of the most likely causes. The digging of deep foundations for large housing estates, office blocks and commercial buildings, will result in a lesser detrimental effect on the family than say, the scene of a road traffic accident or mental/physical abuse.

In recent years I have also found that the planting of genetically modified crops will create these stress lines, as Mother Earth tries to rid herself of this unnatural harvest. In fact, any bad farming practice will produce the same effect. You will also find them leading from hospitals, prisons, care homes, football stadiums and so on.

In most cases they will have been created some way from your home, they follow lines of least resistance, and you might just happen to be the unlucky family having one or more running through your home, the cause of which has no connection to you whatsoever.

When I draw stress lines on my house plan, I use a red pen.

## Dowsing diagnostic questions for stress/disturbance lines:

1. Is the home affected by stress/disturbance lines?
2. How many?
3. Where are they?
4. How detrimental is each one?
5. How were they created?
6. When were they created?
7. Was I or the family responsible for setting any of them up?
8. How long are they?
9. Am I allowed to heal them all?
10. Do I need to heal the source of the line first?

29

# 30. Karmic Problems – Simultaneous Life Trauma

So much has changed in my thinking of how our lives might actually work, rightly or wrongly. And in the next two sections, I will explain how both parallel lives and simultaneous lives may be affecting your life detrimentally.

The dictionary definition of Karma: (in Hinduism and Buddhism) is that the sum of a person's actions in this and previous states of existence, is viewed as deciding their fate in future existences. When I talk to Buddhist friends about karma, they and I know that there it is so much more involved than this rather simple description. There are so many other factors to take into account. But it will do for now as this tends to be the most popular definition. The basic idea is that if you did something bad in a previous life, it will have a detrimental effect on your reincarnation (this life).

But as Tim and I wrote in *Spirit & Earth*, the Earth is a playground, it is here for us, not the other way around. And yes, we are here to learn lessons, but should that mean our mistakes should be carried through to affect our next life? No, I don't believe so. We all make mistakes, and that is simply part of being human, the trick is not to repeat them, and to resolve them within the same lifetime.

I feel that the title 'Simultaneous lives' is perhaps a better way to describe our past, present and future, as we are living all of our lives at the same time but in different dimensions or universes.

Time is only a reflection of what changes in our lives. Man invented the clock in order to control humans. You must be in work at this exact time, it's time to go home, time to have lunch and so on. Einstein said that time is relative, and flexible, and "the dividing line between past, present, and future is an illusion".

So, reality is ultimately TIMELESS.

Non-linear time is a difficult concept to grasp; but you could liken it to a ball of rubber bands. Each band is a whole lifetime, but crosses and interacts with other bands (lifetimes) at many different locations. You could say that the further back the life was, the closer it is to the centre of the ball, with the more 'recent' lives on the outside. This would explain why we are often more affected by events and emotions from our more recent lives than the very distant ones, although if something very traumatic happened, it will reverberate around the ball.

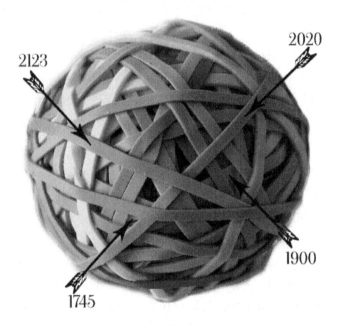

*Time is like a ball of rubber bands, with many crossing points, it is not linear*

It makes sense to me that we are leading all of our lives at the same time. It would appear that the further we progress into the 21st century, the thinner the veil between worlds/dimensions is becoming, making it easier for us to switch from one life to another, albeit only for microseconds. That is when you get that sense of déjà vu, when you know what is waiting around the next corner, when you recognise someone and they recognise you, because in another dimension you have been there just a few moments beforehand.

## Case Study: French Resistance

A good friend of mine had glimpses of a 'previous life' in which she was in the French Resistance during the Second World War, blowing up trains and generally causing mayhem. The flashback that she had was so vivid, that she had heard her name being called, and although it was a male name, she recognised it and the person who called had called out (she was male in that life).

"It wasn't a dream, as I was walking along a path in broad daylight minding my own business when I suddenly felt that I was in France on a dusty road with my resistance friend beside me, I had a sudden compulsion to dive into a ditch and to hide from an enemy troop carrier coming towards us to avoid capture. It did not last long, and no, I didn't jump into the ditch, but the fear was very real just as if I was there. I could even tell you the name of the village we lived in, and my friend's name'."

30

I have had a number of clients since then who have recounted similar experiences, and I have a similarly been affected myself.

## Case Study: An Alchemist

I have been regressed by a very well-known medium and I recalled three of my previous lives, one as keeper of the stones in Avebury, one as an Italian troubadour, and also as a Native American Shaman. Each life was so vivid as I connected to it, I could feel the warmth of the sun or the cold wind, I could hear people talk to me and in several instances could actually converse with them.

Then I went on an in-depth weekend course hosted by Esperide Ananas, a leading light within The Federation of Damanhur designed to look at the ramifications and meaning of a significant 'past' life. How, by learning the lessons from that life, it that would help my progression in this life.

I was based in a small village on the Austrian/Italian borders and during the day I was a skilled artisan, making intricate jewellery and many other artefacts, but by night I had a secret life as an Alchemist. Within my home I had a cleverly constructed trapdoor that was invisible to the naked eye that led down to a cellar where I would meet with several like-minded friends, mixing herbs that we gathered or grown to create medicines for the local villagers, and, of course, experimenting with various chemicals. In those days, if I had been caught, I would have been tortured and killed as heretic or witch.

That was fine whilst I was living alone, but when I fell in love with a local girl, got married and had children, the dynamics changed, I suddenly became responsible for others. Therefore, I closed and sealed the trapdoor and halted all my alchemical work to keep my family safe. Although I adored my family, I yearned to open the trapdoor once again, to get back to the work that I loved, the work that made me happy.

I never did, as my responsibility to the family was too great. I walked over that trapdoor many times during the day and each time I did I got more and more distraught. This unhappiness ate away at me and I died at a young age, around 34.

Why was this so significant? Because I was given a similar choice in this life, and about 9 or 10 years after seeing Esperide, I finally opened the trapdoor, ventured down the stairs and started Dowsing Spirits.

As I was working with this 'past life', I became that person. At the time of the regression weekend, I was still an estate agent and did not have a clue what was in store for me. It was held in Islington, London, and I was living in Surrey. I still remember the drive home on the Saturday night. It took me hours, not because of the traffic, but because I was living that former life, and I was more used to riding a horse than driving a Jaguar. I did eventually get home, but it was a very fraught journey.

I had a very disturbed night and when I did sleep, my dreams were vivid glimpses of my former life, the initial joy of having a family, leading to long periods of unhappiness and depression when I finally realised that I could not continue doing what made my heart sing.

Sunday was when it all came out, the pent-up emotion and sadness. I remember tears rolling down my face as I recounted to the other attendees what I had discovered. I was that unhappy person, I felt everything that he had felt, I had temporarily lived his life.

Looking back on that weekend, I know that I had become him. It was, perhaps, one of those crossing points of time, the ball of rubber bands, when two simultaneous worlds merged together momentarily.

I often think of 'my concurrent family' and send healing to them regularly, to assist them in their life without me in it. To ensure that they have a long, happy and bright life together.

Wouldn't it be amazing if we could all tap into our simultaneous lives, to be able to extract and use their information and experiences to add to our knowledge? I hope that the above story shows that you can. It may take time (if I can use this word) for you to open your mind and to believe. Meditation will help you to achieve this, but you need to be patient.

Eventually you will start to get insights into those lives, and you can ask your guides to help you. Or you can seek out a good medium who could help you on your journey of discovery, opening the doorway to your simultaneous lives.

We need to send healing to these other dimensions, which could then be sent all the way around the 'ball of time'. We could effectively clear our 'collective lives' of detrimental attachments (if appropriate), cut any psychic and physical cords, send healing to their families, and work on their homes. The possibilities are endless.

The healing would likely be reciprocated, can you imagine how effective this could be? The power we could generate by concentrating on ourselves and our many lives for just a few minutes each day. The ripple effect would travel through the space/time continuum.

Another one of Einstein's theories is that there is a fundamental link between time and space. The Universe, for instance, has three dimensions: left and right, up and down, backwards and forwards – plus one time dimension. This dimension he referred to as the space-time continuum.

So, it would seem we have no past, present or future, all we have is now and we could be living hundreds, if not thousands of lives, all at the same time and these lives can overlap with each other.

With the questions below I would suggest that you still view time as a historical concept. It is easier to dowse the time period in centuries, and once you know that information, it is easier to ascertain the problem that we have to heal.

For the healing process to go smoothly, you will need to have the whole story mapped out; from the very first time the physical/mental injury or karmic/dimensional trauma took place to the last, probably this life. You could read through the case studies in *Heal Your Home* as they will give you a better idea on what to look for and how to ask the questions, slowly building up the story of your past/dimensional lives.

It will take time but is so worthwhile. Are you the injured party or the culprit? Have you created the karmic/dimensional debt or is there another guilty party? Is it someone close to you, a family member or work colleague, or perhaps someone that has already passed away?

## *Dowsing diagnostic questions for karmic problems – simultaneous life trauma:*

30

1. Do I have any debts or problems affecting me from a simultaneous life?

2. Do I have more than one problem?

3. Are any members of my family affected?

4. Who?

5. Can I identify in which life it started?

6. Are we counting back or forwards in hundreds of years or thousands? (If hundreds, then start to count from 100 upwards, until the rods move, indicating a century. Then, count in 10s to get the decade, and then from 1 to 10 to get the exact year).

7. Am I living in Europe in that life? (or America, Asia, Africa etc.)

8.  Am I male or female?

9.  Am I a person of ill repute?

10. Have I made a stupid mistake - or was it premeditated?

11. Have I repeated this in any other of my lives?

12. Did I hurt someone mentally?

13. Did I hurt someone physically?

14. Did I kill someone?

15. Can I learn the lesson in this life, to stop the pattern repeating in other lives?

16. Can I heal the any debts/trauma that I have in this life?

17. By working on this life for myself (or members of the family), will it help in this life?

*NB You can ask any of the above questions for each individual member of your family.*

30

# 30a. Karmic Problems – Parallel Life Trauma

A parallel life means that there is a version of you, in this same time period, in the same body, who is living in a parallel or alternate universe/dimension to this one. In all likelihood, there won't be just one parallel version of you, but perhaps dozens. As we saw in the interdimensional place memory section, what happens in these parallel lives can affect us in this dimension, perhaps causing that feeling of déjà vu (a French term literally meaning 'already seen') experienced in a simultaneous life, a feeling that you have been in this situation before.

So, if a parallel version of yourself gets ill, gets divorced (see vows or contracts, section 27) has an accident, moves home, or indeed, gets married, those actions can cause ripples that can affect you in your current dimension.

30a

My favourite illustration of this concept is the wonderful film called 'Sliding Doors'. Written and directed by Peter Howitt, starring Gwyneth Paltrow, it demonstrates the concept of two lives taking place at the same time. One in which she catches the underground train and the other when she does not. I highly recommend it.

Why is it that some mornings you can wake up feeling great, yet the next morning feel like you have the weight of the world on your shoulders, or a bad headache? We could blame modern day stress, but what if the other you, in a parallel life, is going through difficulties, hard times or is just unhappy? Those feelings may be bleeding through the thinning veil

194

and have a detrimental effect on you. And, of course, vice versa, you may be affecting them in the same way.

By determining whether we are being affected by the actions of a parallel self, we can start to clear any detrimental energy that might have come through the veil, sending healing to our corresponding self, and then to protect ourselves from receiving further disruption from the other dimensions.

## Case Study: Another Adrian

I am now a house healer, having been an estate agent and before that an antique dealer. Now let us picture a different Adrian, one living a parallel life, who did not follow his heart and is still running his estate agency business.

He wakes up one morning feeling massive regret that he did not take Andy Roberts' comment seriously when he said, 'You can do this, you can be a healer, and by the end of the year you will be shifting some very big stuff.' I can only imagine how he must be feeling, stuck in a commercial world that is sucking him dry, knowing that he has missed his chance to live a more holistic and spiritual life, something that he has wanted for so long.

Can you imagine the unhappiness, day in day out, stuck in a job that he is growing to hate, the waves of his despondency moving through the ether? And as this happens, I feel that our subconscious minds can link, 30a or at least receive an echo from these other lives.

We therefore need to be aware that our other selves can be in turmoil, suffering all sorts of physical, mental and spiritual anguish. So, whenever we carry out a healing on ourselves, and this should be a very regular occurrence, we need to focus not just on this life, but all of our parallel lives.

This healing will work both ways, what you send out you will receive, the healing will move back and forth between all of our lives, each dimension then adding to its energy. Can you envision what an amazing impact that will have on all our lives?

## Dowsing diagnostic questions for karmic problems – parallel life trauma:

1. Do I have any problems affecting me from a parallel life?

2. Are there problems affecting me from more than one parallel life?

3. What is the problem?

4. Can I send healing to the parallel version of me, and clear the effects of the problem?

5. Can I protect myself from being affected by this parallel life?

30a

# 31. Detrimental Implants

Anything alien placed into our body could be called an implant, including life-saving devices like a pacemaker. Each pacemaker will have its own individual vibrational energy that may or may not harmonise to the person it is planted into. Each will have been manufactured, packed, transported to a hospital, unpacked, stored for future use, and then finally taken to the operating room where a team of surgeons and theatre staff will carry out the necessary surgery.

At each step of the way it is liable to pick up detrimental energies, starting from its manufacture to finally entering the human body. The emotions of all the people handling it, the nurse who places it into the surgeon's hands, and of course the surgeon themselves. Each will leave an imprint, all potentially detrimental to the recipient.

So, we need to bless and send healing not just to the patient, but also the pacemaker, making sure that it is clear of any detrimental energy patterns. This goes for anything that is surgically placed into our body: stents fitted to the heart, anything involving a heart by-pass, any joints being replaced whether the hips or knees, metal pins holding together a broken bone due to an accident and so on.

There have been recent reports of chips that can be inserted into your wrist, which you then wave over a contactless payment machine to pay for goods. It feels like a futuristic concept, disposing of the need for us to carry cash and credit cards around, but this type of technology has been with us for years.

Some silicon enhancements have also proven to be very unhealthy. Although they can do wonders for self-confidence, in the long term they need regularly checking on to make sure that they are still safe.

I feel it is a good idea to make sure that you do not have anything implanted into your body that you are unaware of. A quick dowse, asking the question, will give you the answer, and do not forget that we are only looking for detrimental energy patterns, so, if they aren't detrimental to you leave them alone.

I admit that I have not found anything suspect, although there are many stories circulating of microchips being injected into your body via vaccinations, whilst others have reported receiving them from certain food stuffs or fizzy drinks.

UFO abductees have also reported implants in their bodies, sometimes they have been able to feel them under their skin. So that buzzing in your ears might not just be tinnitus, it could be feedback from a brain implant, so dowse and check. Again, ask if it is detrimental as you might find an etheric angelic download has similar affects.

Implants can be energetic as well as physical. Whilst being attuned to Reiki, symbols are inserted into your aura, if the ceremony is not carried out correctly then the symbols can be easily be corrupted, and the wrong ones implanted. Sometimes a re-attunement may be necessary.

If you are working on family or friends, you may find it better to hold back some of the information that you have found. Implants can be rather a sticky subject to explain and can cause upset, concern and fear.

## Dowsing diagnostic questions for detrimental implants:

1. Do I, or any of the family, have a detrimental implant? (Spiritual, ET, physical etc.)
2. How many?
3. Was it through a surgical procedure?
4. Do I need to clear the implant in my body?

5. Is it the material that they are made with?

6. Or the emotion of the surgeon/doctor and nurses in the hospital?

7. Where are they attached?

8. When were they implanted?

9. Do they need to be healed or worked on to rid them of any detrimental energies?

10. Can they be neutralised or harmonised today?

11. Do I have a corrupted Reiki symbol in my aura?

12. Do I need to be re-attuned?

13. Has the wrong healing symbol been given to me?

14. Can I heal the problem myself or do I need someone else's help?

31

# 32. Toxic Lines

I am finding fewer toxic lines affecting homes as the years go by, but when dowsing a house in the USA recently I came across one affecting a client's house. I was not expecting it and was about to move on to the next question when my dowsing rod moved in a positive response to the question.

Through my questioning, I determined that although it was connected to the fracking taking place in the area, it was linked to the actual process, not the fissures caused. It was the water, sand and chemicals that were injected into the shale at high pressure, to create the gas that is then collected. It was the toxicity of the chemicals used that created the line, essentially detrimental pollution in the soil.

This had set up a toxic line that ran through the ground for many miles. They are often allied to fault lines as that is the easiest way of allowing the detrimental energies to dissipate. My client's home was directly in the path of this very toxic line. The youngest son had developed a breathing problem and the daughter a persistent cough.

They felt something was wrong, because before they had moved to the area both children were healthy and showed no signs of any problems. I worked on the area where they were fracking first, sending healing not only to the site, but to the men involved in the process, continuing up the food chain to the CEO and the main board of the company. I finally cleared the toxicity from the line and harmonised the energy patterns.

Hopefully by including all the people involved in the healing, they may begin to understand that what they are doing is irrevocably harming the planet. The intention and healing, was of course, sent to them with unconditional love.

When detailing these lines, I draw them in pink.

## Dowsing diagnostic questions for toxic lines:

1. Is there a toxic line affecting the house?
2. How many?
3. Where are they?
4. How detrimental is the line?
5. Is it detrimental to both men and women?
6. When was it caused, what date?
7. Why was it caused?
8. Can it be healed?
9. Do I need to heal it at source first, then the home?
10. Can I heal it for other people too?
11. Do other layers exist?

32

# 33. Chakra Alignments and/or Blockages

It is almost impossible for all your chakras to be in balance all the time, especially here in the western world, due to the stresses and strains of everyday life. We are emotional beings and one or more will always be out of kilter, even if only slightly. Despite this, it is good practice to consciously balance your chakras as often as possible.

Each chakra is an energy centre of the body, allowing external universal life force to enter and then flow through our physical form, energising us.

In *Heal Your Home*, I went into detail about the seven main chakras that most healers work with, but as you can see from the psychic protection method at the beginning of this book, I now regularly work with ten chakras. They are located in the feet, knees, base or root (around the perineum), sacral (just below the navel), solar plexus, heart, thymus (aka the upper heart), throat, third eye or brow and finally the crown (top of the head). There are also a range of colours associated with these centres as I have detailed in the psychic protection method.

Humans all work in very different ways, some will approach daily life from the head and some from the heart, and because of these differences, we will all use very different chakras during the course of the day. A person working in a complementary therapy field will use more of their crown, third eye, thymus, heart and solar plexus chakras, whilst those in business will be more likely to utilise their base, sacral, solar plexus (for energy), throat and crown.

All will be spinning away, but not in balance, because we are using or nurturing some more than others. Perhaps when we sleep, they may start to settle and balance, but then as we start to dream the equilibrium is upset once again.

It is therefore better to ask that all chakras are working at the appropriate maximum capacity, or as close to maximum as we are allowed to get, whilst carrying out a particular job or task, and then to then settle into normal living levels once finished or are finally back at home.

It is easy to forget that our chakra points, (apart from those at the base of the spine and the crown of the skull), are at the back as well as at the front of the body. Therefore, if there is a blockage or misalignment, check both the back and front of each chakra, as a blockage can occur just on one side.

## Dowsing diagnostic questions for chakra balance/ blockage:

1. Are any of my chakras out of balance?
2. Which ones? (Remember front and back)
3. Can a flower remedy rectify the problem?
4. If not, do they need individual healing?
5. Which one or ones?
6. Can wearing a specific colour bring the chakra into balance?
7. When did this happen?
8. Are any of my chakras blocked?
9. Which ones? (Remember front and back)
10. Can a flower remedy rectify the problem?
11. If not, do they need individual healing?
12. When did this happen?

33

# 34. Anything else affecting the house and family (in garden/grounds or close by)

This is a general catch all question that I ask when dowsing the plan of my clients' home. All it requires, to begin with, is a yes or no response. If you get no, then breathe a sigh of relief as it saves asking a lot of further questions. If you get yes then you need to work out what the problem, or problems, might be.

In *Heal Your Home*, I called this chapter 'Anything Else Running Through The Site' but I feel that the new title is the better, because it reminds you to ask if there is anything detrimental in the garden or grounds that might be causing the family problems. It also includes anything that might be running just outside the boundaries.

It could be an ancient trackway, a funeral path, an old tunnel, a cave or a Roman/Pagan road. Many of these can have some form of detrimental human emotion attached and potentially a number of spirits (both human and animal). There may be a ley or other forms of energy lines that don't actually touch or run through the house, but their detrimental patterns may just reach and cause the family some health problems.

## Case Study: Neighbours

I became aware of this problem whilst working on a home in Wigan. I had dowsed the house and family, drawn up the plan, typed the report and discussed my findings with my client. Then came the feedback and I began the fine-tuning exercise, checking to make sure that all was well, that any layers that might have appeared were worked on and healing sent.

All was going well, but I felt that something was missing or perhaps something that I had not yet uncovered. Every now and then I come across a 'learning house', a property that has me digging deep, metaphorically speaking, trying to work out what the new detrimental energetic pattern is, how it affects the family and whether it can be healed and harmonised.

This is where the new questions come from. These situations can be exasperating, but ultimately, once solved, it will be for the benefit of all my future clients, and indeed anyone reading this book.

So, I had asked the question 'Was there anything else running through the site?' and got a no response. That was quite right as there was nothing else, however when asked if there was something 'outside' their boundary that was affecting them in a detrimental way, I got a yes response.

It turned out that there was a powerful energy channel running through the house across the lane and it was adversely affecting the family who lived there, but none of the detrimental energies were actually penetrating my client's house, so I was still a little mystified.

This is where it gets interesting. I spoke to my client and asked him how he and his family got on with the neighbours living opposite. His answer was quite short, only four words initially, 'They are a nightmare'. It all boiled down to the car parking situation. Which was quite logical and, in many towns, probably an everyday occurrence. But this particular situation got more involved the deeper I delved.

The energy channel was not actually harmful to my clients; however, it came in at -7 in detrimental effect for the family opposite. Living over something that powerful would have a big knock-on effect, as they probably wouldn't be sleeping and this would naturally lead to a shortness in temper, irritability, feeling ungrounded and generally just not being happy with the world.

This irritability would erupt every now and then and the only thing that they ever complained about was car parking. This would upset the whole neighbourhood as they would park their cars too close to others,

34

blocking them in and then not answer the doorbell to move them. They would also bend windscreen wipers and break off wing mirrors. Everyone knew it was them doing the damage, but it was always done after dark so that no one could prove it.

The damaging effect on my client was not directly to do with the energy channel, but the ramifications of its effects on the family opposite creating a detrimental impact on them. It was not a psychic, physical or psychological attack, but a combination of all three.

I asked Upstairs if it was appropriate for me to carry out a clearing and healing on the energy channel and got a yes response. I also sent appropriate healing to the family as they very much needed the help.

Since then, everything has calmed down, there is the occasional blip, but overall, the family has been very quiet, and no cars have been damaged since.

Working out a problem will certainly test your dowsing and questioning skills; in fact, you may find there are several problems linked together, but hopefully the questions below will help.

Try to find a date to begin with, this will give you somewhere tangible to start. You then need to know your history or carry out some research on the internet.

## Dowsing diagnostic questions for anything else affecting the house and family (in garden/grounds or close by):

1. Is there anything else affecting the house and family (in garden/ grounds or close by)?
2. Is it a line or perhaps a spirit that needs helping?
3. What century does this anomaly date back to?
4. Is this BC or AD?
5. Has it contained human/animal traffic over the years?
6. Is it running above or below the ground?
7. Is it man-made or natural?
8. Is it a footpath, bridleway or ancient road?

9. If none of the above then is it a cave, tunnel, mine, drain, cable?

10. Is it or was it used daily, weekly, monthly?

11. Has anyone been hurt here?

12. Has anyone been killed?

13. Is there anyone buried here or close by?

14. Are there any spirits to help go to the light?

15. How detrimental is this problem to me (the family, client)?

16. Can it be healed?

17. Can I carry out the healing or do I need someone to help me (energetically)?

18. Is the detrimental energy coming from a nearby ley or earth energy line?

19. Is there anything else for me to find?

20. Are there any layers to clear?

34

# 35. Fabric of the Building

Previously, when issues with the fabric of the building arose during a home healing, I found it was because the stones or bricks had come from sites where great turmoil had occurred, and the materials had retained that detrimental patterning and needed clearing. For instance, the rubble used in the foundations of the building might have come from a derelict psychiatric hospital, factory, or sacred site.

For example, many houses in Avebury have large pieces of Sarsen stone, from the Circle, that were broken up and incorporated into the walls of the houses.

But it has come to my attention over the years, that the fabric of a building, whether commercial, residential or retail, can absorb detrimental energies from the people within them, especially during times of hardship, crisis and upset.

The lockdown in 2020 and 2021 due to the Covid-19 virus was a major trigger point, and the outflow of fear, uncertainty, stress, concern over money, an unhappy workforce, or threat of bankruptcy, will all have left their mark. Not just on the people, but also on the walls, floors and ceilings too. Not to mention on the furniture, computers, coffee mugs, pens etc.

Some of the detrimental energy will be picked up when you ask about 'Human Emotional Energy Areas' (see Section 17), but these tend to be

35

found within the building, but we need also to consider the actual fabric of the building, the bricks, mortar and plaster. In fact, any materials that may have soaked up the anguish of a collapsing company or a failing relationship and the emotional stresses involved.

During much of the 2020 and 2021 lockdown period, thousands, if not millions of people spent many months staring at the same four walls and in many of the cities and larger towns people were often too afraid to leave their homes for fear of catching the virus. Understandably, this confinement saw a big rise in mental and physical illnesses, and not only were people eating and drinking more, but they were also unable to exercise.

All this pent-up emotion has to go somewhere, and sitting for hours in a particular chair, for instance, could lead to the creation of a power artefact. In the same way that spending most of the day moping in bed could. So, these items will all need individual healing.

But most of the angst and torment can have soaked into the very infrastructure of the house. If you decided to sell, chances are a potential buyer would enter your home and straight away walk into a thick blanket of detrimental emotional smog. Which is not likely to result in a sale.

It is therefore a particularly good idea to carry out a weekly clearing on your home of any emotional upset and anxiety that the family may have created. If you are selling, this should be done before any prospective purchasers come to view.

## Dowsing diagnostic questions for the fabric of the building:

1. Is there anything detrimental about the fabric of the building?
2. How detrimental is it?
3. Is there more than one area affected?
4. Is it above the ground?
5. Is it below the ground?
6. Does the detrimental energy come from the earth?
7. Is it man-made?

35

8. From when does it date?

9. Can it be healed?

10. How many layers are there?

11. Does it involve an act of violence?

12. Are any spirits involved with this energy?

13. Is there a build-up of detrimental human emotional energy that needs to be cleared?

14. Do I need to clear this every day/week/month?

15. If I do not, could it be detrimental to a sale?

# 36. Anaesthetic Traces, Inoculations, Vaccinations, Heavy Metals

## Anaesthetic Traces:

In the past, traces of anaesthetic used in an operation could be found months (or even several years) later in our body. It could result in the person feeling lethargic, suffer from insomnia, brain fog and so on.

Modern methods are far kinder and more efficient, the anaesthetic disappearing from our bodies within a few weeks of the operation, so rarely are the affects detrimental for long periods of time.

A simple question is all that you need to ask: 'Am I, or any member of my family, suffering from any long term, or detrimental, affects caused by anaesthetic'? If the answer is no, then move swiftly onwards.

## Inoculations and Vaccinations:

If you do any research on the internet you will find as many pros as there are cons when it comes to inoculations and vaccinations. Though these two things may appear to be the same, and they have similar meanings, they do differ slightly and this, apparently, is mainly historical.

Vaccination: is the introduction of a vaccine (an agent that resembles the disease-causing microorganism) into the body to help the immune system develop protection from a disease.

Inoculation is a method of artificially inducing immunity against various

36

211

infectious diseases.

Much of the controversy around vaccines relates to the use of Thiomersal (a mercury-based chemical) as a preservative in many of the vaccines available globally. This is due to it being linked to the rise in Autism, ADHD, and immune system dysfunction.

According to medical sources, Thiomersal is no longer used, but many parents are still uneasy and unsure about the long-term effects that vaccinations could have on their children.

There will be, I am sure, a vaccine developed to halt the spread of and develop an immunity to the Covid-19 virus and this is going to be worth billions of dollars to the large pharma companies. In an altruistic world it should be sold at cost and given free to the people, but I doubt that would happen while there is a profit to be made.

This is a difficult area to work on as most people in the developed world have had countless injections over the years, whether for diseases like measles, mumps, tetanus, or in preparation for travelling abroad. And the older the person is, the more likely that they will have received a vaccination containing Thiomersal.

So, checking for any lingering detrimental effects from previous vaccines is essential, as is setting the intention that any vaccine received in the future only has a positive effect, and any detrimental side effects are cleared quickly.

## Heavy Metals:

I still find certain heavy metals affecting some of my clients, but this is becoming rarer as the years go by. The two easiest and most common heavy metals absorbed into our bodies are mercury and lead. Nowadays, there is less mercury used in amalgam fillings for our teeth and very few lead pipes still bringing water into our homes.

But the fear is still there, as is the worry over aluminium cookware, the health risks of Teflon in non-stick pans, and the chemicals and metals contained in tap water.

36 Allyson and I were lucky enough to be given the most wonderful water

filter/purifier made by Berkey. It has been in use for a year or so and we have been so pleased with how the water tastes. The water in North Yorkshire is not too bad, but the chemicals added still taint the flavour and smell. Once the water has filtered through the Berkey system, it is both drinkable and has no distinguishable odour. It also makes a great scum free cup of tea.

Also be aware of the toothpaste that you and the family use. Both Allyson and I are great advocates of fluoride free toothpaste made by Aloe Dent and it comes in many flavours including Charcoal, Triple Action, or Whitening. I suggest that you carry out your own research regarding the effects of fluoride in both toothpaste and water.

## *Dowsing diagnostic questions for anaesthetic traces, inoculations, vaccinations, heavy metals:*

1. Does my body have any detrimental anaesthetic traces?
2. How detrimental is it?
3. Can it be cleared or healed?
4. Any detrimental traces from vaccinations?
5. How detrimental is it/are they?
6. What vaccination was it?
7. What age was I when I had the vaccination?
8. Is mercury the problem?
9. Can the problem be cleared or healed?
10. How long will it take?
11. Do I need to seek out a specialist to help?
12. What kind of specialist?
13. Will I feel better once this problem is clear or healed?
14. Do I have a problem with heavy metal levels in my body?
15. Which heavy metal or metals is/are responsible?
16. At what age did this exposure occur?
17. How did it happen? (Diet, work, etc.)

36

18. How detrimental is it?

19. Can it be cleared?

20. Do I need to seek out a specialist for help?

21. What type of specialist?

22. How long will it take?

23. Will I feel better after the treatment?

24. Is it beneficial for me to filter drinking water?

25. If I don't, how detrimental is the water?

26. How detrimental is fluoride to me and the family?

# 37. Parasites

I sometimes find, after I have started working on a house, that one or two members of the family succumb to mild flu-like symptoms with aching bones, feeling tired, stuffy nose, no energy and a fuzzy head, but this would usually only last for a few days and then disappear. These are similar to the effects of parasite die-off.

As you begin to heal the home, it will likely disrupt the parasites in your body or your family's bodies, even if you are doing this from a distance. The healing vibrations can trigger changes in the body, acting rather like a purging agent, detrimentally affecting the parasites, and as they die, they release neurotoxins, heavy metals and viruses into the body and this, I feel, causes the flu-like symptoms.

Just to clarify the point, it does not happen to every client, but interestingly I have noticed that those that it has affected often suffer from IBS (Irritable Bowel Syndrome).

## General signs and symptoms of parasite infestation include:

Headaches

Brain Fog

Bloating – acid reflux, constipation, and diarrhoea

General aches and joint pains

Fatigue

Skin problems including rashes

Emotional disorders including anxiety and depression

Cravings for food and alcohol

Stuffed up nose and aching sinuses

Insomnia

Weight gain and also weight loss

## So, where do these pests come from?

Swimming pools

Drinking Water

Lakes and ponds (contaminated water)

Various foodstuffs (if not washed properly)

Restaurants and takeaways (especially when abroad)

Soil

Blood

Sexual Contact

Pets

Mosquito Bites

There are many methods that you can use to eradicate the harmful parasites in your body including a visit to your GP for a test. If it comes back positive for parasites, they will prescribe the correct medicine to take. However, the NHS normally only tend to test for the 'big guys' as Kate Chaytor-Norris explained to me, that is unless you ask your doctor specifically to look deeper. Therefore, your tests may come back showing nothing untoward in your gut because the smaller parasites were not picked up on.

Or you can go the more natural route using herbal remedies, but I would very much recommend you consult a good naturopath or homeopath first before doing anything.

Carrying out a general gut cleanse, before a full eradication treatment is recommended, as it will help reduce the symptoms of die-off, which can be quite acute, but this does depend on how badly you have been affected in the first place. Eating lots of organically grown greens and drinking plenty of filtered water will certainly help the process, and you need to make sure you take the correct doses of any remedy you are prescribed.

Going the natural route may take a little longer than using mainstream medicine, but it does tend to be kinder to you and your body. Do be patient as it can take many months for the little blighters to be fully eradicated from your body, but when you get the 'all clear' you will be feeling so much better.

Kate, who has written a real 'go to' book called '*I Wish My Doctor Had Told Me This*', also explains that the parasites can develop a Bio-Film around themselves, like a protective coating, and you may have to take a variety of remedies before you are clear.

Kate added 'After the treatments are over it is a good time to start replenishing the good bacteria in your gut by taking a good Pro-Biotic and eating fermented foodstuffs such as sauerkraut, kefir, and kombucha'.

I must thank Kate for steering me in the right direction and recommend her invaluable book which is available via her website www.nutritionyorkshire.com or on Amazon.

## *Dowsing diagnostic questions for parasites:*

1. Do I have any detrimental parasites in my body?
2. How detrimental are they?
3. How long have I had them for?
4. Did they come from contaminated food?
5. Did they come from contaminated water?
6. Did I get them from one of my pets?
7. Can they be removed through healing?
8. Should I see a specialist to clear them?
9. A homeopath, nutritionist or doctor?
10. Will I feel better once they are cleared from my system?
11. Is my IBS caused by parasites?
12. Is my depression caused by parasites?

13. Is my weight gain/loss caused by parasites?

14. Are my food cravings the result of parasites?

15. Can my alcohol cravings be attributed to parasites?

# 38. Off-World Interference, Psychic Attack, Psychic Cords

A psychic attack coming from another human is a reasonably well understood and known concept, but this section is a whole new ball game and the subject needs to be treated very seriously. When it appears that you are being psychically attacked, but you cannot easily find the source, it could be that an Off-Worlder is the culprit.

Let me explain what an Off-Worlder is.

When I found my first psychic cord that was not connected to another human being, my mind automatically went to the Elemental Kingdom as we co-exist with them on this planet, sharing our living spaces, gardens etc. But they were not the source and I apologised to them unreservedly.

So, the next step was to ask whether this attached silver thread came from an E.T. (Extra-Terrestrial Being), I got a slight movement on my dowsing rod, not the normal yes response, it was more like 'keep going and ask the next question'.

So, I did:

*Is there life on other Planets? Yes.*
*Within our Solar System? Yes, but not physical beings like us.*
*Are we looking more at Micro-organisms and bacteria? Yes*
*Is there Extra-Terrestrial life in physical form? Yes.*
*Do they look like us? No.*

*Have they been to our planet in that form? Yes, but not for hundreds of years.*

*Are they still visiting us? Yes.*

*In physical form? No.*

*In a psychic/clairvoyant way? Yes.*

*Can they link into everyone that way? No.*

*Does there need to be a weak point for them to do so? Yes.*

It seems that if our aura, the natural electro-magnetic field surrounding our body, is strong and fully energised, they cannot psychically penetrate it and attach a cord.

*Once the cord is attached is it detrimental to us? Yes.*

Why are they doing this? From my questioning, I found that they want to learn what it is like to be human. Earth is a very special and unique place, and there is nowhere else like it, anywhere. These beings do not experience any form of emotion, love and hate is unknown to them, as is envy, jealousy, wonderment, and passion. By linking to a human through a psychic cord, they can experience all of these emotions. But this interaction comes at a price for the person that they have linked to.

It can cause a sudden onset of a headache that never goes away, a loud and continuous buzzing in the ears (rather like tinnitus) or a static-like sound in the head - a feeling that someone is 'messing with your brain'. The person affected could also begin to act out of character, feeling that they are being pushed to do something that they really don't want to do, like drinking too much, or a sudden desire to release their emotions, at an improper time.

These cords are rather like 'communication cords', similar to a two-way radio. Therefore you will need to find out which chakra or chakras they are linked/attached to as this is where the cords will need to be cut.

This psychic link or cord (there can be several, so do ask how many there are) needs to be severed as soon as it is discovered, and a block put on any further attacks. Psychic protection will then become imperative to stop the cords from being reattached, as it not only clears your body, but also the auric field (the shield) surrounding your body, keeping you safe from further attack.

I will often put my client into a mirrored pyramid (see healing section for details) for a few days, just to safeguard them, and provide added heavyweight protection.

## Simultaneous/Parallel Life cords

There can also be psychic links coming from human beings living in our simultaneous or parallel lives, so do ask the question and deal with them accordingly (see the healing section).

There was a programme on TV back in the late 60s called *The Time Tunnel* where two men called Doug and Tony got stuck in a time loop, travelling backwards and forwards through time.

They faced all sorts of dangers, from attacking dinosaurs to the Crusades, on the first space mission to Mars, experiencing first-hand the eruption at Krakatoa and a lot of hazards in between. Now either of them could have been killed at any stage, but wouldn't it be good to have this time travel experience without the fear of dying? Well, that is what I believe is also happening.

I believe that in an advanced society, sometime in the future, we have developed a way to link, psychically, into another human being living in a different dimension.

But doing so comes at a price, not necessarily for those in the future, but for the poor person they have psychically linked to. Causing the onset of a bad headache, looking in the mirror and not fully recognising themselves, irrational behaviour, and/or potentially try to change their appearance, but not understanding why.

I have come across these links many times now and have cut them. I admit to holding some of my findings back from clients, as I feel that it can appear way too far 'out there' and difficult to explain in simple, down to earth terms. So, I put the information down as a simple human psychic attack.

## Dowsing diagnostic questions for off-world interference, psychic attack and psychic cords:

1. Am I or any of the family suffering from ET or off-world interference?
2. Who is affected?
3. How long has this been going on?
4. Is there a reason why it happened?
5. How detrimental is this interference?
6. Is there a cord or link that needs to be severed?
7. Where does this cord/link attach i.e. which chakra or organ?
8. Once cut, does the person need extra protection?
9. How long for (days, weeks, months)?
10. Do I need to check again to makes sure the link has not re-attached?
11. If so, when (days, weeks, months)?
12. Is there anything else that I need to know (problems with aura etc.)?
13. Are there any cords or links attached, psychically, from a different dimension?
14. How many?
15. Can I cut them all now?
16. If not, then when can I cut the next tranche?
17. Does the person now need psychic protection?
18. How long for?

# 39. Off-World Lines

I first came across these lines when teaching my 'The Secrets of Healing Your Home II' course in France. One of the ladies who had come to the UK to take the first of my 'Secrets' courses, lived in France and at the conclusion of the weekend said, 'Why don't we hold the second course in my home, it can be part work and part play'. So that is exactly what we did, several months later.

Six of us gathered for a very interesting weekend. The house turned out to be a wonderful Chateau and of course, it needed some healing before we could start, luckily, we had a few days in which to do this before the course started.

Everyone was quite used to dowsing their floorplans by this stage, so we continued where we left off in England. Part way through we asked the question 'Is there anything else affecting the house and family (in garden/grounds or close by)', I saw Rob's (one of the attendees) dowsing rod twitch indicating yes.

I do like it when this happens, as it keeps me on my toes. We ran through various questions to find out exactly what Rob had found and it went something like this:

*Have I found anything like this before? No.*

*Is it earth energy based? No*

*Is it man-made or caused by human interaction? No.*

*Does it have energy running along it? Yes.*

*Both ways? No.*

*How long is the line? I started counting and reached approximately 8 to 9 miles.*

*Does it run along the surface of the Earth? No.*

*How far beneath the surface is it? Around 45ft to 50ft*

*Is it naturally occurring? No.*

*So, has this line been manufactured? The rod moved slightly to say that I was on the right track but not yet there.*

*Are we looking at a pipeline or conduit? The rod twitched again as if to say, 'get on with it'.*

*Is it solid? No.*

By this stage my brain was starting to hurt, and I felt that I was running out of questions to ask.

A good time for a coffee break (I do love French coffee) and time to 'phone a friend', a spiritual one, hoping for some divine help.

So, to recap. We had some sort of pipeline, but not a pipeline as it wasn't solid but still contained some form of energy that ran in one direction and it wasn't related to the Earth, around 8 to 9 miles in length and located 40 – 50ft beneath the ground.

I asked Rob was there anything nearby that might have some sort of pipeline running to it or from it?

'Yes', he said, 'a power station and it isn't far from where we live, in fact I work there.'

That gave me the next question.

*Does the 'pipeline' originate from there? No.*

*Does it lead to the power station? Yes.*

*Is it drawing something from the power station? Yes.*

*Is what it is doing harmful to us? Yes.*

*Harmful to the planet? No.*

224

*If the pipeline is not solid could it be dimensional or holographic? Yes.*
*Is it of this world? No.*

The upshot of these questions was that this particular holographic 'pipeline' was created back in the 1950s by Off-Worlders, designed to run beneath the ground and extract 'in secret' an energy that was a by-product of whatever created the electric current produced by the power station.

39

This was then transported back to their home world for use there and they had been carrying out this operation for many years, undetected. So, the detrimental line running beneath Rob's home turned out to be a very exciting find. Since then, I have discovered a number of others around the country.

The reason they are detrimental to us is not what the pipeline contains but the frequency used to develop and maintain the holographic pipeline. Its vibrations can be very disruptive to us humans and animals, something the Off-Worlders were totally unaware of. They certainly did not mean us any harm.

Now we had discovered the pipeline I needed to work out how to go about fixing the problem without interfering with its operation, and this, I found out, was something that the Off-Worlders were very worried about.

Several weeks after my French trip I had booked to teach a 'Secrets' course in Welwyn Garden City to a group of very sensitive ladies. They were all good friends and held regular meditation and healing evenings and it was during one of these meetings that they received a very stern warning about my forthcoming visit.

It went something like this:

'You are going to be visited by an hombre shortly, he has unearthed something that was never meant to be discovered and he is the only one who knows about it. Tell him that if he talks about it to anyone, we will kill him and the people who he has revealed his information to'.

I was not sure what to think when they told me, it is not every day that you get a direct threat from an 'alien' species. I was not sure whether to

225

be excited that I had found something that no one else had discovered or terrified of what they might do to me.

I decided to be slightly circumspect which I think the ladies were grateful for. I purely mentioned that I had discovered these off-world lines and that they can be detrimental to us and told them 'if you ever dowse and find one let me know and I will deal with it for you'. Better for them to be safe than sorry.

That seemed the most satisfactory way of dealing with the problem and for the next year or so, when teaching a course, I kept the description as brief as possible and carried out a healing on any lines that attendees had found.

However, it still niggled me, after all, I live here on this planet, they do not. I also wondered how they would organise the hit…

Sometime later, I was working on a large house in Devon in conjunction with a very talented medium and mentioned to her about the warning I had received, she tuned in and questioned her main guide, his reply was 'They have a big ego, don't take them seriously'.

Having worked on many of these lines since, I now know that they were being melodramatic, and do not have the ability to end my days. They were obviously worried that I was going to disrupt or bring an end to their operations, but that was never my intention, I just wanted to ensure that no harm came to my clients and their families.

Hopefully, they now know that we have the ability to work on these lines, to harmonise the detrimental harmonics given off and balance the vibrational energy patterns, without disrupting the flow or cause them any anxiety.

## Dowsing diagnostic questions for off-world lines:

1. Is the house affected by any off-world lines?

2. If so, how many

3. How detrimental is it to the family?

4. Am I allowed to heal them as directed by Adrian's harmonising method?

226

5. If not, is Adrian able to help me do so?

6. When were they created?

7. Where does it run from and go to? (You will need to map dowse this, the information isn't necessary for working on the line, purely for your own curiosity).

8. Is the energy being extracted to help life on another planet/ dimension?

9. Will harmonising the line be beneficial to me and my family?

# 40. Detrimental Planetary Rays

This isn't something that I have comes across in very many client's homes (as I write this book). However, it is one of the 'mop up' questions that I ask, just in case it is the key to unlock the final door to what ails them.

I have been finding that for the last few years we are being affected by rays coming from the other planets in our Solar System, and also beyond. So, why is this happening?

This is due, I feel, to the many space probes that have been launched over the years, the Voyager series in particular. Voyager 1 was launched in the late 1970s and is still going, now into interstellar space, the furthest any man-made object has ever gone.

As we see the spectacular close up, high-definition photographs of our neighbouring planets, they are drawn further into the human consciousness and as this happens the more of an effect they will have on our psyche. This effect is not always harmful, but when we are healing our homes and family, we are trying to ascertain what is detrimental to us, so it will be the rays affecting us in a destructive way that we need to dowse for.

So, how do these planetary rays affect us? Our Earth is under constant bombardment from solar winds, clouds of fast-moving electrons, protons, and ions, generated by the sun. They are responsible for creating the phenomena known as the Northern Lights (Aurora Borealis) and the

Southern Lights (Aurora Australis).

These streams of charged particles, released from the sun's upper atmosphere, can create havoc with our communication systems, especially during prolonged periods of solar flares, and because we are also electro-magnetic beings it can have similar effect on us, to a greater or lesser extent. All of these energies are bouncing around the planets, rather like a pin ball machine, some reaching us on Earth.

40

A photon is a particle of light, and when these photons are "absorbed" by a molecule, they gain in energy. But that extra energy can make the molecule unstable, causing it to release the energy that has built up. The direction that the photon then moves in is completely random, and it can also be absorbed by a denser atom. The energy will eventually escape as the photons move away from the surface.

It does depend on where we are living on the Earth as to which planets may affect us and when. They may be visible to you in the night sky, but do not forget that they can be there during daylight hours, even though you cannot see them.

I know that the moon is not technically a planet and is a satellite of the Earth, however the effects can be very much the same. At the height of the full moon there are more photons being bounced around and absorbed by us, which often produces detrimental effects in people, such as insomnia and heightened emotions.

I know that there are people who feel that this is a fallacy, but there is a noticeable increase in the number of telephone calls that I receive as we enter a full moon period. I keep meaning to leave a message on my answer machine saying, 'Please be aware that we are once again entering a full moon period, hormones will be raging, and emotions will be intensified'.

Each planet vibrates at different levels and these frequencies can be detrimental to us, and cause sleeplessness, hormonal changes, irritability, lack of energy or a feeling of lethargy. Unlike the full moon, the planet can be in the sky for several weeks and the harmful effects are therefore prolonged.

There can also be a lot of psychic energy coming from the planets too and we need filter out the good and the bad. Mercury, for instance, is a very psychic planet and its energies can have an effect on us especially when it is in retrograde. All the planets moving around our sun travel in the same direction but have differently shaped orbits, so it can sometimes appear that a planet is moving backwards in the sky, referred to as retrograde. Mercury retrograde is not a good time for communication, it can feel like you are walking through treacle. It's certainly not a good time start a new project, and relationships can be strained.

## Dowsing diagnostic questions for detrimental planetary rays:

1.  Is a member of the family or the home detrimentally affected by any planetary rays?
2.  Who?
3.  If so, is it a planet or moon within our own solar system?
4.  Which one?
5.  If not, is it is one of the well-known constellations?
6.  When did this start?
7.  Is it intermittent (if so, is it daily, weekly, monthly, seasonal)?
8.  Does it affect any members of the family physically, mentally or psychically?
9.  If so, who is it?
10. How does it manifest itself (tinnitus, headaches, irritability)?
11. Can I carry out a healing on the rays?
12. Does daily psychic protection help?
13. Can I protect the house?
14. If so, how do I do this?
15. Am I being affected by any psychic energies coming from the planets or stars?

# 41. *Technopathic Stress*

Technopathic Stress is the detrimental energy given off by underground or overhead electric cables, power lines, mobile telephone masts, tetra masts, general household wiring, energy-saving light bulbs, Wi-Fi, or smart meters, microwave ovens etc. Even a gas or water main can cause health problems.

The changes in lighting have been illuminating (sorry) with the widespread use of LEDs (light emitting diodes). They have revolutionised how we can light our homes safely. They produce a steady light without flicker, unlike the earlier and widely used long-life energy-saver lightbulbs and fluorescent bulbs which contained vaporised mercury.

LED bulbs come in several different shades, warm white, brilliant white, daylight and universal light, they also come in different colours. It is good to use a warmer white LED in your bedrooms, a blue spectrum light in your task room/study (to simulate daylight), and the living room should be more into the red spectrum which will help you to relax and unwind.

The term "Dirty Electricity" is becoming a widely used to refer to many electronic appliances, energy-efficient lights, and other devices that run on electricity in our home or workplace. They can produce a high frequency whine, buzz, or cause lightbulbs to flicker (now linked to epilepsy in humans and animals). Some people are more susceptible than others to these effects and could experience symptoms such as headaches, heart palpitations, nausea, or brain fog.

It is becoming more common because many of the devices in our home no longer use straightforward AC voltage electricity, instead the current is manipulated in order for the television or modem to operate and this causes spikes and erratic surges of electrical energy.

The electricity, therefore, is no longer harmonious and these frequency variations can combine to form complex and potentially harmful electromagnetic fields.

The best way to avoid many of these problems, especially when we are asleep, is to switch as many appliances off as you can, including televisions, mobiles phones, tablets and modems. And during the day, switch them on only as you need them. It is good practice not to have your mobile phone in your bedroom whilst you are sleeping. If you do, make sure that it is turned off. Because as you relax your body is at its most susceptible to the harmful radiation given off by your mobile phone, it will certainly interrupt the depth and quality of your sleep. Try leaving it in the kitchen at night and see what a difference it makes.

There are many people out there who do not believe that electro-magnetic fields can be healed, cleared or blocked by intent or prayer. Humans and animals are electro-magnetic beings who derive benefit from healing, so why can't the same be said for man-made EMFs? I have found that energy healing and psychic protection can indeed safeguard you from the harmful effects of technopathic stress and is particularly useful when it cannot be avoided.

Awareness is the key here. If you have walked into a modern office building and start to feel off-colour, your head suddenly feels fuzzy, or you are a little dizzy then the chances are you are affected by the man-made energies in the building i.e. technopathic stress. So, before you enter the front door intentionally increase your protection by visualising a bubble of white light around you, which should help.

## 5G

Many scientists and doctors are concerned about the detrimental side effects of the new 5G network that is being rolled out as I write this (in 2021). But the government have found no identifiable risks while running its first tests of the technology. Though I guess that they would say that, wouldn't they?

Only time will tell with regards to 5G, my personal opinion is that we will see many more people suffering with diseases such as Alzheimer's and dementia, some with brain tumours and other illnesses, which makes me fear for the next generation.

My dowsing tells me that this will be the case although I have not yet come across anything detrimental affecting any of my family, friends, and clients. But it is still very early days, and I am sure it will not be long before I do.

For those of you wishing to delve deeper into how electricity affects us I can thoroughly recommend Arthur Firstenberg's (a scientist and journalist) book entitled *The Invisible Rainbow: A History of Electricity and Life* in which he links flu pandemics with the adoption and mass installation of electrical technology worldwide.

## This is a part of the introduction to his book:

'We live today with a number of devastating diseases that do not belong here, whose origin we do not know, whose presence we take for granted and no longer question. What it feels like to be without them is a state of vitality that we have completely forgotten.

'These are the diseases of civilization, that we have also inflicted on our animal and plant neighbours, diseases that we live with because of a refusal to recognize the force that we have harnessed for what it is.

The 60-cycle current in our house wiring, the ultrasonic frequencies in our computers, the radio waves in our televisions, the microwaves in our cell phones, these are only distortions of the invisible rainbow that runs through our veins and makes us alive. But we have forgotten. It is time that we remember.'

## Smart Meters:

We also have the Smart Meters to contend with in our homes and they are more commonplace now than when I wrote *Heal Your Home*. In fact, we have one in our current home. Allyson tried to get it taken out, but our supplier said that it couldn't be done. The reason being that there are no old-style meters to re-install, as soon as they are taken out, they are scrapped, and no one is making new ones. So, we are stuck with it.

But to safeguard our health I have carried out a healing on the meter, asking that it is cleared of anything that may be detrimental to us, harmonising its energies to work with us rather than against. Ironically, I have not yet managed to reduce my bills.

Why are smart meters detrimental to us? They connect to a 'secure national network' and send out short bursts of microwave radiation at various times during the day to keep your supplier up to date with your power usage. They operate in a very similar way to your smart phone and there are major concerns about the long-term health risks of the use of them especially for teenagers and younger children whose brains and bodies are still developing.

Long-term exposure to microwave radiation is also known to be harmful as it disturbs all the natural processes in our bodies. After all, look at what it does to food when you use a microwave oven. A lot more power is needed to cook your food, but the process is similar to your smart phone, and for those whose only means of communication is via a mobile device, the prolonged use will have health side-effects in the future.

## Classic symptoms of over exposure to microwave radiation:

Headaches and Dizziness
Short-term memory loss and brain fog
A fuzzy head
Feeling irritable and a short temper
Aching joints
Insomnia and general sleep disorders
Digestive problems
Heart palpitations
High and low blood pressure

## Hybrid Cars:

In the last few years, hybrid cars (those using a combined petrol and electric motor system) have become more popular on our roads. Complex engineering that is heralded to save our planet from exhaust fumes (and other chemicals) that are produced by a pure internal combustion engine.

But are there any detrimental consequences to us as humans when we enter and sit for several hours at a time in a car full of this electronic wizardry?

Over the last twelve months, a number of clients have emailed me to say that since buying a hybrid car they have started to suffer from bouts of nausea and headaches when travelling for any distance. It didn't matter whether they were driving or a passenger and wondered if it was anything to do with the workings of the car.

And guess what I found?

Yes, it is.

Just like any other forms of geopathic stress, our bodies will react to these external electro-magnetic impulses, but some people are more susceptible than others. The electric motors emit extremely low frequency electromagnetic fields, and this can be a cause for concern.

The jury is out at the moment, some experts are saying that these EMF's are completely harmless to us whilst others are saying that there will be long-term consequences, and that the body cannot safely sit in these EMF's for long periods of time.

My suggestion is to bless your car and, in fact, anything you buy or bring into your home should undergo a similar process. This might feel simplistic but saying the following whilst holding or touching the object

'I ask that all detrimental and inappropriate energies that are affecting me and my family, including any electro-magnetic fields, are taken away and disposed of in an appropriate fashion. I also ask that my car (or any other object) in now flooded with light and love leaving it in peace, balance and harmony. I ask that the healing takes place not only in this dimension but all other dimensions that are similarly affected.'

See if that has made a difference, and in the case of hybrid cars, I would also suggest protecting yourself and family before entering the car and setting off on your journey.

## *Dowsing diagnostic questions for technopathic stress:*

1. Is there detrimental technopathic stress in the house?
2. Where does it come from?
3. How detrimental is it to the family?
4. Should the Wi-Fi be turned off at night?
5. Can it all be healed by intent?
6. Can these energies all be harmonized to work for the good of the family?
7. Does an amethyst crystal help with the EMFs from a computer?
8. Is the microwave detrimental to our health?
9. How detrimental is the food once cooked in the microwave?
10. Should I use the microwave at all?
11. Do we have any dirty electricity in the home?
12. Which appliance or appliances does it come from?
13. It is good switch off all unnecessary appliances at night?
14. How detrimental is my mobile (cell) phone if left on my bedside table at night?
15. If I leave it downstairs will I sleep better, deeper?
16. Are any of the lightbulbs in the house detrimental to the family?
17. Are electric blankets detrimental to my health?
18. Is a hot water bottle a better choice?
19. Is 5G going to be detrimental to me and my family?
20. How detrimental will it be to each individual member?
21. Is the smart meter detrimental to me and the family?
22. Is Bluetooth detrimental to you and the family?
23. How detrimental is my smart phone when switched on?

24. How detrimental is it when I am making a call?

25. Can I heal any of the detrimental energy coming from my smart phone?

26. Am I or any member of my family detrimentally affected by the energies in our hybrid car?

27. If so, can we carry out a clearing on them?

28. Will the psychic protection method help us to dissipate the energies?

41

# 42. Human Interference Lines

I am still finding these human created lines, but only intermittently. They are human-created disruption lines, set up mentally and mechanically to affect other people in a detrimental way – rather like white noise, but with no sound attached.

The energies that they produce interfere with our brain patterns. Rather than sending and receiving clear impulses to and from the body, they become scrambled and are not easy to interpret. You may experience buzzing in your ears, headaches and balance problems; you may also feel rather nervy and restless. These intent lines disrupt our lives. They spread melancholy and negative thoughts, leading to disturbed sleep patterns and irritability.

The more that I study these lines the more I find that they are set up with dark commercial intent, and that there are studies of the short-term effects of harmful radio waves sent in pulses over a short distance, to observe how it affects people along its path.

I believe this is with a view to developing a weapon (pulse cannon) that can be used against humans, leaving buildings undamaged. It may sound like Science Fiction, but that is what I feel is being experimented with.

After a few weeks or months of radiating, the beam is switched off and then the doctor's surgeries in the locality will be monitored for any patients being treated for any unusual illnesses. This is so they can prove to a government what they have developed works, and actual figures could then be produced. The statistics will prove its effectiveness.

Only time will tell if I am right but do check to see if you or your family and friends have fallen victim to such electronic interference.

## Dowsing diagnostic questions for interference lines:

1. Is the home affected by an interference line?
2. How many?
3. Is it/are they detrimental to me and the family?
4. How detrimental is it?
5. Is it created by human intent?
6. Is it the result of a machine?
7. How does it affect me and the family?
8. How long is the line?
9. Where does it come from?
10. Has it been set up on purpose?
11. Can it be healed or blocked? Which one?
12. Can I heal/block it?

42

# 43. Fracture Lines Caused by Fracking

Fracking has become a hot topic since I wrote *Heal Your Home*, rather like 5G, and it is still very much in the news. Here in the UK, fracking has been happening for years, but without public knowledge of the practice and its harmful effects. It began earlier in the US, with hydraulic fracking starting in 1949.

Fracking creates problems for humans, and I am beginning to see the detrimental effects that it has on my clients, their families, and houses. The effects produced are similar to fault lines. But whereas fault lines are naturally produced by the spinning of the Earth, these fracture lines have been caused by human greed.

These fractures cause lines that can run many miles away from the actual site. These ruptures may be minor, but they have been the cause of several earthquakes in areas that have never been affected in the past. The harmful effects of these lines come from both the human element (upset and emotion) as well as the detrimental energies caused by the damage done to the Earth.

As these harmful energy patterns run along the fracture line, they can affect large numbers of families and their homes along the way.

We must also look at the harm that the fracking method is causing to the planet. Water (often millions of gallons) is pumped underground at a very high pressure, full of very toxic chemicals, into the shale in order for gas to be released. The harmful effects are obvious, not just to the planet, but to us and animals.

## Case Study: Fracking Fissures

The first time that I picked up a detrimental problem from fracking was when working on a client's house in Frome, Somerset.

I know there has not been any fracking close to Frome, but the problem had come from about 50 miles away. It was not the actual fracking that had caused the problem, but the testing that they had carried out initially to see if the operation was going to viable.

Whether it came from a test drilling site or they had carried out seismic surveys, it had caused minute fissures in the earth, spreading out from the epicentre in many different directions. It felt as though Mother Earth was trying to diffuse the local devastation.

How did I pick up this line? The question at the very end of my checklist is one of the most interesting and often the source of a new query, 'Is there anything else for me to find that is detrimental to the family?' I got a yes response and picked up on a harmful line running directly through my client's home. I just had to work out what it was and how it was created.

Is this a naturally produced line (as in earth energies)? I got a slight yes so needed to continue with my questioning, I was partly there as nature had been involved in creating the line.

*Has the detrimental energy been mainly caused by man? Yes.*

*Is it some form of earth disturbance? Yes.*

*Does it differ from a stress line? A slight twitch from the rod.*

*Is it caused in a similar way (as in earth disturbance)? Yes.*

*But it is different? Yes.*

*Has it been produced in a very specific way that I have not found or seen before? Yes.*

In the weeks building up to this new find, I had been researching fracking finding out what the extraction process consisted of and why people were so upset about it. So, my next question was:

*Has it been caused by fracking? No.*

*Is it anything to do with the fracking process? Yes.*

*Has it got anything to do with the testing or exploration that they are doing? Yes.*

Finally, I had narrowed it down. It was not being caused by fracking per se, but the testing and drilling had caused small fissures to appear, leading directly from the epicentres of the various exploration sites in the area. Now I knew what caused the detrimental effect to my client, all that I had to do was work out what form the healing would take to help both them and Mother Earth.

I started with the personnel involved in the testing site, before sending the appropriate healing to the workforce, and then moving upwards via the foremen, management, CEOs. I finished by sending healing to all the various test sites, and finally along all the cracks and fissures that they had created.

## Dowsing diagnostic questions for fracture lines caused by fracking:

1. Is the home detrimentally affected by fracking?
2. If so, how detrimental is it?
3. Was it the testing that caused the fractures?
4. Or was it actually the fracking process?
5. Where did the fracking or testing take place (map dowse the location)?
6. Has it created one or more lines or fractures?
7. Is part of the problem airborne (gas or chemicals escaping into the atmosphere)?
8. Can it all be healed?
9. Is some of the energy contained in the lines caused by human emotion?
10. How much is earth linked?

11. How long is the line?

12. Is it okay for me to send healing to the human element of the problem?

# 44. Harmful Frequencies

**These sounds can consist of both high and low frequencies:**

High Frequency Sound: a high-pitched whistle, a scream or a child's voice.

Low Frequency Sound: any form of bass noise (such as the thump you hear from a car sound system), a drum, a man's deep voice and thunder.

**Then we have the following:**

High Frequency Noise: Crashing symbols and birds.

Low Frequency or Background noise: road traffic, aircraft, wind turbines, air conditioning units, industrial and garden machinery, and wind (air movement).

All of these sounds can be detrimental to us as humans, and sometimes you can identify where the noise is coming from and other times not. For instance, we had a tinny whine in the house recently, it was very quiet, but it was there, constant, and extremely irritating. I thought that it was me for a while, then I asked Allyson if she could hear it too.

She could hear it, but also did not know where it was coming from, she had tried to find it, but could not discover the source. We both listened and it seemed to be coming from the hall, she checked the various smoke and $CO_2$ detectors, but they were not to blame. I got a chair and climbed up to listen to the meter cupboard, but it was not that either. I finally pinned it down to the telephone answering machine. So, I switched it off for a few seconds and then back on, and finally the sound stopped.

It hadn't been very loud, and it wasn't there for more than 7 or 8 minutes, but it had been extremely irritating, and I had found it difficult to concentrate on the healing work before me. Can you imagine how debilitating it would have been if it had been louder and I had been unable to do anything about it?

Which is how it would be living next door to an engineering works, with a constant high-pitched whine being created by machinery, or the constant hum of motorway traffic.

Sounds can be conducted through rock strata, underground water or streams, and crystalline structures. You may also have turbulence caused by a nearby windfarm, as well as the noises created by the huge blades turning in the air.

*These noises and sound waves can produce the following:*

Headaches

Disturbance in our natural balance leading to giddiness and nausea (rather like sea sickness).

Tinnitus

Fatigue

Inability to concentrate

Blurred vision

Insomnia

Dizzy spells

## Case Study: The M5

The first time I came across this issue was when Alan, an old friend, called me asking for help. He and his wife had been to stay with friends in the West Country and he had become quite ill whilst there. His symptoms included dizzy spells, the sudden onset of a headache, lack of concentration and unable to sleep for any length of time. He felt a lot better once he got home and within a few days he was back to normal, but he was very curious to find out what had caused him to feel the way he did whilst there.

He gave me their address and sent me a location plan; the house was situated on the outskirts of a small village surrounded by countryside. It looked idyllic, but often when you dig deeper, you can find that 'snake in paradise', the one little thing that spoils the ambience and tranquillity.

In this case, it was the M5 motorway.

This was how I narrowed down the problem:

I spoke to Alan and asked if the family he had stayed with were all in good health. He said no, they always seemed to be suffering with something, always had coughs and colds. The wife always looked very pale, the children were listless, and the husband very stressed. They had relocated from London, seeking peace, quiet and fresh air, but as Alan said, 'They all seemed to be healthier when they lived in the city'.

I checked the house, and it was reasonably clear. There were a couple of spirits to move on, some earth energy lines, spirals and water veins to heal, but nothing that really stood out as the major culprit. I could not find anything there to explain why Alan felt the way he had.

So, I asked the question:,

*Is there anything else that is detrimental for me to find? Yes.*

*Is it a new problem for me to solve? Yes.*

*Is it earth energy related? No.*

*Man-made? Yes.*

*Does it come from within the house or village? No.*

*When working out how far from the house it originates, are we working in feet or miles? Miles.*

*How many miles? Under 10 miles? No. Under 20 miles? Yes.*

*I then started counting upwards from 10 until I reached 19 and the rod moved.*

*Are we looking north, south, east or west? West.*

I opened the OS (Ordnance Survey maps) program on my computer,

246

found their village and traced a line 18 miles roughly towards the west. As my eyes reached the M5 motorway the rod moved indicating that was the location of the problem affecting both the family and Alan. I just needed to find out what it was.

The first that I thought of was pollution, the sound of traffic and/or fumes. But could either of those affect a family living 19 miles away? Yes, was the response.

*Sound? Yes.*

So, I called Alan and asked if he had heard the motorway when he was there, he had not and said that the family had been concerned about that very issue making sure that the house was far enough away not to be bothered.

*Was the traffic sound audible? No*

*Was it a vibration coming through the air? No.*

*Was it a vibration coming through the ground? Yes.*

*Ah ha, now we were getting somewhere.*

*It is being transferred along a fault line? Yes.*

So, we had a low frequency sound or vibration travelling along an anomaly or weakness in the earth straight into their house. It may not have been audible, a lot of low frequency sound is not, but their bodies were picking up on these detrimental vibrations.

Our body is similar to a tuning fork, left alone it vibrates at a perfect pitch until something touches or interrupts it, then it goes out of tune.

I then had to sit down quietly to ponder how I was going to carry out the appropriate healing on this newly found problem. You can find my method in the healing section. Several months after I carried out the healing, Alan went back to stay at the house and suffered no ill effects. He also reported that the family were much healthier and happier.

There are a number of 'active noise control' machines now on the market, they emit a sound wave at the same scale as the original noise, but inverted, this interference cancels out the original sound, creating a new wave.

They are using the same technology in cars to help cancel engine and road noise, in offices to help to mute background sounds in meetings, and also in homes that are affected by traffic.

I feel that we can do exactly the same but using intent rather than a machine.

## Dowsing diagnostic questions for harmful frequencies:

1. Am I, the family or home affected by harmful frequencies?
2. Is it from high frequency noise/sound?
3. Is it from low frequency noise/sound?
4. How detrimental is it?
5. Is it created within the home?
6. If no, then is it within close proximity?
7. If no, how far away does it come from?
8. Does it come via the air?
9. Does it come through the ground, as a vibration?
10. Does some form of manufacturing process cause it?
11. Traffic, wind turbine etc.?
12. Can it be healed?
13. Can the family, be shielded/protected from its harmful effects?

# 45. Guardian of the Site, Spirit of Place or Home

You will find a lot more in-depth information on this topic in my second book, *Spirit & Earth*. My co-author, Tim Walter, and I had many long discussions about each of the characters and what they represent to us as humans, how they affect us, where we can find them and how to communicate with them.

There is also more information contained in *Heal Your Home*, but I will summarise it here, so you know what you are dowsing for.

Guardian of the Site: Every sacred site has a guardian attached to it. They are a custodian, a necessary and fundamental part. A location does not have to be considered (by us humans) to be holy or sacred to have a guardian, as to them, all places on the Earth are. Which is why we need to check our homes for them, even if it they haven't been built on what would normally be considered a sacred area.

The guardian tends to be a devic being, coming from and being part of the Earth. They are very protective of their territory and can easily take offence should anyone behave in a disrespectful manner. This, of course, goes for minor transgressions like dropping litter, or not tidying up after your dog, to the major upset of someone building houses on an open field which they have protected, and where they have resided for hundreds of years.

We need to treat them carefully and with deference, it is better to have them on your side than actively working against you. The guardian of the site is perhaps best considered as the 'front of house' whilst the spirit of place is more like 'management' and therefore will have less contact with humans.

## Spirit of Place:

The spirit of place tends to be made up from the core element of a site, the physical and spiritual. The Romans referred to them as Genius Loci, the protective spirit of place.

A site like Avebury will have various guardians, one for each segment of the site (split by the road system) but only one spirit of place, they are the overseer of the whole. They are the steadying influence, holding much of the sacredness and memories of the site within its boundaries.

They adopt an umbrella view of the site, unlike the guardian who is more confined and territorial. The spirit of place concern themselves with the welfare of their sacred site and are very protective and proactive towards maintaining the sanctity and purity of the whole.

They get very concerned and upset when any human activity disrupts or alters the sacredness of the site, which in turn can easily disturb the natural pattern of the environment. They let their displeasure be known physically, with a shove in your back when there is no one there, the sudden onset of a headache, feeling very uncomfortable, unsettled, or afraid.

## Spirit of the Home:

The atmosphere or feel of a property is created by combining all the human emotional patterns that have been left behind by anyone visiting or living in the house. The full range of emotions, from joy and happiness to upset and trauma, are all absorbed into the walls, ceilings, and floors, making the house feel very comfortable and homely or cold and uninviting.

It is a direct reflection of us, just as our personality is manifested in the colours of the walls and the furnishings. We can create an intimate, tranquil, and homely atmosphere using earth tones or a more modern environment, using striking vibrant colours and shades. The decoration echoes our tastes, interests, and values.

The emotions and decor combine to give each house a different feel, to create an individual sacredness or sanctity. To me, this is the spirit of your home. Not a living being, but more of an ambiance with each room feeling different. You want the bedrooms to feel calm and unhurried, the living room to be relaxing, the study to be lively and inspiring, and finally the kitchen to be the powerhouse.

Each room can be programmed to be exactly what you want it to be, each with its own unique atmosphere. First, they will need to be cleansed of all past emotional patterns and then you can introduce the new energies, giving each room its own healing space or 'hot spot' as appropriate.

I have worked on many homes over the years and I have never yet found one that doesn't need some form of healing, much of it based around the detrimental emotions left behind by others, and so spiritual hygiene is therefore important, as it keeps the spirit in your home.

45

## Dowsing diagnostic questions for site guardians and spirits:

1. Does the home have a guardian of the site?
2. Does the home have a spirit of place?
3. Does the house have a spirit of the home?
4. Is each one happy?
5. If not, how detrimental are they to me and the family?
6. Are they detrimental to the pets?
7. Can they be placated by intent or actions?
8. What do I need to do to make them happy, i.e. plant a tree, etc.?
9. Should I talk with them regularly whilst in the garden?
10. How long have they been there?

# 46. Elementals in the House and Detrimental Pathways

If you have read my first book, then you will see a slight change in the title with the addition of Detrimental Pathways. This inclusion will be explained as you read through this section.

Elementals or nature spirits are wonderful beings, the true workers of the world. They vibrate at a lower level than us, therefore are rarely observed, but often we can sense them, especially when walking through a remote glade of trees, or by a quiet stretch of water.

They toil away relentlessly in our gardens, ridding them of pests (if we ask), looking after new shrubs and plants that need nurturing and encouraging new growth everywhere. But if they get trapped or lost in our homes, they can create a number of different problems, depending on what type of the elemental they are.

A water elemental hiding in your pipes can cause blockages and leaks, they can affect your boiler and make unusual noises in the plumbing system.

Earth elementals can be easy to upset, they like routine and hate change. Especially when we build a house on a path they have been walking for many years.

Fire elementals are the easiest nature spirits to see, but if they get trapped, they can also cause your household boiler to malfunction, or in fact anything to do with heat in your home can be affected.

If air elementals get trapped in the home, they can disrupt the natural flow and movement of the air, suddenly making a room feel stuffy and airless. A candle blowing out for no reason, smoke that was rising up the chimney one minute suddenly blows back into the room when there is no wind outside or disturbing your family pet as they blow into its ear.

If you wish to see fire elementals, you ideally need a fire pit, lots of wood, a box of matches or a lighter and a mobile phone, then wait for darkness to fall. Get the fire going, building it up with the logs, until you have good flames rising from it, then start taking photographs with your mobile phone or iPad. Keep snapping away, take as many as you like, then once finished start scrolling through, looking for patterns in the flames. If you're lucky, you should start to see recognisable shapes and patterns, those are fire elementals.

Some will have recognisable shapes, for instance, I have taken some amazing pictures over the years including a baby dragon rising from my fire pit, a griffin, a phoenix (literally rising from the flames), and the best of all was the Devil complete with a pitchfork. You can also ask for the fire elementals to reveal themselves to you as you take the photographs, they normally oblige.

Our ancestors understood the land, they would talk to the fairies, imps and gnomes, and they in return would communicate with us. Try sitting quietly and tune into the local spirit, giving thanks for all they do for us. Your garden will start to bloom in many different ways.

## Case Study: Disgruntled Nature Spirits

A client of mine, Britt, lived in Norway but had a holiday home in Sweden. The location looked delightful, but the house had a problem that would not go away. It was built over a path used for generations by the Nisse (in Norwegian or Tomte in Swedish), solitary creatures that are easily offended, extremely irritable and quick to temper. They are part of the natural world and are very protective of farms, the land, buildings, and animals.

In both Sweden and Norway, they are associated with the Winter Solstice and the Christmas period. They look very much as we picture a dwarf here in the UK, short in stature, with long white beards and wearing a red pointed hat.

I had worked Britt's home in Norway initially, but was asked to look at her holiday chalet, because she wanted to sell it and although there had been a number of people looking at it, no offers had been forthcoming, which was very unusual. It was a popular resort and houses rarely stayed on the market for long, she was keen to get it sold before the winter set in.

There had been niggly problems with both the plumbing and electrical systems over time. Both would fail intermittently however the source of the faults could never be traced. When working on the house I had found a few resident elementals and I had helped them move back into nature, but they were not the main culprits and had only played a very small part in the problems.

I felt that there was something more for me to find but was not prepared for what it was.

*Is the problem found in just one location in the house? No.*

*Does it run through the house? Yes.*

*Some form of line that can be traced and mapped out? Yes.*

So, I did.

I worked with my crystal pointer and rod, I found where the line entered the house and where it came out, marked it in black and then had to find out what caused it.

*Is it man-made? No.*

*Earth energy related? No, I also included energy channels, fault lines and other lines, they were all a no.*

*Is it an old footpath? The rod slightly moved indicating I was on the right track.*

*Was it used by man? No.*

*Elementals? The rod moved slightly.*

*Is 'a form of nature spirit a better definition'? Yes.*

Due to my experience with elementals, I assumed it was a Troll Path but

254

when I asked the question, I got a no response. I admit, at that time, not knowing anything about Scandinavian nature spirits, whether they were the same as we have here in the UK, so I asked my client to see if she could help.

She did and told me that they were called Nisse or Tomte, armed with that information I went online and did some research on them.

They, like our own nature spirits, do not like change and someone building a house over their well-trodden path was both insulting and downright rude. They were certainly not happy about it and did all that they could to disrupt the energy patterns in the house, detrimentally influencing the electrical and water systems, as well as being able to alter the atmosphere within the home.

I asked if there was a guardian of the site and got yes. So, I tuned in and asked if I was allowed to divert the pathway around the house. There was a slight pause, and I then received a rather reluctant yes. I certainly did not want a disgruntled guardian on my hands so I quickly added 'and I will also divert the path away from all other houses that have been built over it, disrupting the flow'.

46

The suggestion was well received, so that is exactly what I did. First, I cleared away any detrimental energy patterns and emotion that had been created or left by the builders and subsequently the nature spirits, asking that the pathway be divert from each of the offending houses that had encroached or been built on it.

Once that was done, I then had to ensure that the house was also cleared of all detrimental energy patterns that had been created. From what I was told, during my feedback emails, is that the atmosphere quickly changed inside the house, it became lighter and brighter, the musty smells had gone (I hadn't been told about those) and there were no further problems with either the electrics or plumbing system.

I often think about those little fellas, they have added to my knowledge and understanding of how nature spirits work and that a building, in the wrong place, can have such a major impact on their lives and, of course, ours too.

## Elementals in our body:

I was asked some time ago whether it was possible for us humans to ingest elementals. I admit that it was not something I had ever thought about, so I dowsed the question and got a yes response. I then had to investigate whether a) If we did, were they detrimental to us? b) How did they get there? and c) Could they be easily removed?

It does seem that in 99% of the cases, ingesting any form of nature spirit is harmful to us. They are not life-threatening, but they can disrupt the natural functioning of our body. Their lower vibrations can cause our body to start acting sluggishly, we then cannot process our food correctly, leading to digestive problems, lack of energy and so on.

So, how did they get in?

It really depends on which of the elemental groups they belong to and I want to add that this is a rare occurrence, finding one or more within your aura is far more commonplace.

Water is obvious as we have to drink it to survive, but you won't find them coming out of your cold water tap in your house, that is treated with chemicals and they wouldn't survive. It is more likely to occur if you drink water from a river or stream, a natural spring and so on.

An earth elemental could enter if you have eaten any vegetables grown in the ground and not washed properly. Again, it is unlikely to be on any food that you have bought from a supermarket as they have, more than likely, gone through a cleaning process that is harmful to elementals. Therefore, organic root vegetables are more likely to have an earth elemental attached, however if you wash them correctly or boil/steam them you will be safe. We always eat organic and ask that if any elements attached that they leave and move back into the garden.

Wind/air elementals can enter with the breath, though I would say that if you spend most of your time at ground level then there is no need to worry as they tend to stay in the higher air streams. However, if they are disturbed by a hurricane, for instance, they can be swept down to our level. Taking a deep breath on top of a mountain can be a little risky, but most try and avoid being sucked in, preferring to remain free.

46

Fire can be put down to inhaling smoke, anything from a cigarette and cigar to a bonfire and BBQ, sitting around a fire pit can also be a little hazardous, just don't get too close. Anything that is burning can have a fire elemental attached, although more likely if wood is the combustible material used. Coal is also a natural product of the earth but because it is underground it is less accessible and you would rarely find a fire elemental attached.

## Dowsing diagnostic questions for elementals:

1. Are there any trapped elementals in the home, garage, outbuildings or cars?

2. How many?

3. What kind of elementals are they?

4. How detrimental are they?

5. Are they attached to anyone (human or animal), within their aura or body?

6. Is it okay to move them into the garden?

7. Should they be moved further away?

8. If in the garden, will they be detrimental to my pets?

9. Are there any detrimental elementals in the garden that need relocating?

10. Should I talk to them whilst in the garden before I start work, cutting the grass, etc.?

11. Are there any further issues, caused by the elementals, that need to be dealt with?

12. Is the home detrimentally affected by a nature spirit pathway?

13. If yes, can it be diverted?

14. Do I need to divert it from other people's homes as well?

15. Do I need to enlist the help of the local guardian of the site?

16. Before I divert the pathway, do I need to carry out a healing on it?

17. Do any of the nature spirits need help before you do the above work?

18. Have I, or any member of my family, ingested an elemental?

46

19. Is it still affecting me or a member of my family?

20. Which of the elementals is it?

21. When did this happen?

22. Why did it happen?

23. Can they easily be removed?

46

# 47. Tree Spirits

Most trees have their own guardian, referred to as a tree spirit and they are similar, in many ways, to the elementals described in the previous chapter. They are there to protect the tree and help it thrive.

Just like the elementals, they vibrate at a lower level than us humans therefore as not easy to see but with time and patience you can often spot them moving around, from branch to branch, however they do spend much of their time on the main trunk of the tree.

Like elementals, tree spirits can easily become trapped in the house, and when they do, they can be detrimental to the humans residing there, rather like having an angry wasp buzzing around. They can disrupt the natural flow of your home, upset your sleep patterns and cause chaos with your pets. They are nature dwellers and are not happy outside their normal environment.

Once found they will need to be coaxed outside and a new home found for them.

## Case Study: Not a hugger

It was at the time when I was running the Earth Energies Group for the BSD (British Society of Dowsers) and I had organised a weekend meeting near Newbury in Berkshire. I arrived the day before the event and had some time on my hands, so I got in the car and toured around the local villages, getting a better feel for the area.

In one hamlet, I spotted an interesting old church, pulled the car over, switched off the engine, grabbed my dowsing rods, and opened the gate. There are always intriguing and complex earth energies patterns to be found in churchyards, but what immediately caught my attention was a magnificent and very majestic sycamore tree.

It was big, round and imposing. Instantly you knew that it was undoubtedly the guardian of the church and its grounds. I walked towards the tree, wanting to measure the extent of its auric field but as I got closer, I began to feel very uncomfortable.

There was an air of menace, it felt just like a psychic attack. My head began to hurt, and I felt dizzy.

Then I heard the voice.

I had never heard a tree talk, but this one did, and I got the message loud and clear. I was shocked, a) because it spoke to me and b) because of the language that it used.

'Don't you come any f***ing closer'. I stopped and looked around, because at first, I thought it was a human voice, but no one was there.

Then I heard 'You can look, but you had better not touch me.'

I looked at the tree and it seemed to bristle, almost defensively. 'Is that you speaking to me?' I asked the tree out loud, thankful that no one was there to hear me.

'Who did you think it was?'

I wasn't really sure what to say to that, but as they say, 'flattery gets you everywhere' so I replied 'You are a magnificent tree and I couldn't help but admire your stature'. (Once an estate agent always an estate agent.)

'I am the guardian of the tree and the tree is the guardian of the church and grounds.'

I looked at the tree and could see a slight shimmering about 20ft up the main trunk which I figured was the tree spirit.

I asked that it show itself to me and it moved, I wasn't able to see any real shape to the tree spirit, but I am sure there are people that can.

It transpired that both the spirit and the tree were getting fed up with people walking up to them, and without asking permission, wrapping their arms around the trunk, giving them a big hug. It was, as far as they were concerned, very disrespectful and intrusive. I had to agree, as I am sure that I would feel the same way if a total stranger came up to me in public and gave me a hug.

I respected the boundaries and went no closer, thanking them both for explaining the sudden and rude outburst that I had received when I first got there, I tried reassuring them that when humans hug trees they are only doing so with the best of intentions, got in my car and left.

It is a good idea to check, before you cut a tree down or trim its branches, that it does not have a spirit attached. As the tree goes through the trauma, the tree spirits can easily become dislodged or displaced, then can start to cause similar problems to trapped elementals or nature spirits.

If the tree is being cut down, ask the tree spirit to transfer itself to another tree locally, one that is without its own guardian, to dedicate itself to the happiness and wellbeing of its new home.

47

If you haven't got a tree in your garden or one nearby it might be a good idea to go and buy a shrub from your local garden centre and then hold a dedication ceremony, encouraging the tree spirit to move to your new purchase. Do check before you buy, to make sure that it has not already got its own tree spirit.

Also, if you are out on a walk and see a tree surgeon trimming a tree or even cutting it down, for whatever reason, be sure to help the tree spirit, if there is one, move to another tree.

## Dowsing diagnostic questions for tree spirits:

1.  Is there a misplaced tree spirit in the house?
2.  Is there a misplaced tree spirit in the garden?
3.  What kind of tree spirit is it i.e. oak, spruce, elm, yew, etc.?
4.  Where it is?

5. How detrimental is it?

6. Can I help in relocating the tree spirit?

7. Would dedicating it to a specific tree help?

8. Is there a tree in the garden that is suitable? (if not, go to the next question)

9. If I purchase a new tree, and plant it in the garden, then dedicate it to the displaced spirit, will that appease them?

10. Is it beneficial for me to hug a tree?

11. If so, which one?

12. Should I ask permission first?

13. Does it need any healing work carried out?

14. If so what? This could be reducing its auric field to match the new outline of the tree. If it had lost a branch during a storm or had been cut back by a tree surgeon, the original outline of the tree would still be there. The aura would still follow the outline of the missing limb, by shrinking the aura to envelope the tree helps it energetically.

15. As a final check, do ask if the tree or tree spirit needs any further help or healing?

47

# 48. *Animal Spirits*

When any pet or animal passes over, in most cases, they will move naturally to the light. They do not get affected by guilt, fear or lack of worth. But they can be held back by the grief of their owners or if they died suddenly, they may not be aware that they have passed over, especially if they have been 'put to sleep' by a vet. A cat may well have stayed behind to comfort its grieving owner, a dog may feel that it is still rounding up the sheep and a horse is still galloping around with the rest of the herd.

So, just as human beings get stuck on the earth plane, so do animals.

48

All spirits, humans, and animals, that have not gone to the light will be detrimentally charged - it cannot be helped as they should not be here, it is unnatural. They will be vibrating at a disharmonious level to us, but through no fault of their own. It is the same for humans that have had their journey interrupted; they need to go to the light to continue their evolution.

If they do not, their soul cannot progress.

I remember receiving an email many years ago from a rather disgruntled gentleman, who had read my view of this, and said that his dog, who had died some 10 years ago, was always with him and helped him during his healing sessions. He wanted to know how she (the dog) could possibly be detrimental to him.

I wrote back to tell him that she had already gone to the light and had returned to him in pure spirit form, to help him with his healing and provide companionship. But if she had not gone to the light first, then she would not have been able to help him at all, no earth-bound or discarnate soul could.

## Dowsing diagnostic questions for animal spirits:

1. Is there a displaced animal spirit in the home?
2. How many?
3. What type of animal are they?
4. How detrimental are they?
5. Are any of them past family pets?
6. Am I allowed to move them to the light?
7. Will they go willingly?
8. Do they need someone to help them go across?

48

# 49. Animal Created Stress Lines

This is a question that I have recently added to my checklist, after finding an unexplained and anomalous line running through a client's house, not far from where I live in North Yorkshire.

## Case Study: Animal trauma

Whilst working through my checklist, I just had a feeling that there was something else I needed to find, something that I hadn't come across before and I racked my brain as to what it might be. When dowsing the plan, I asked if this anomaly could be viewed as a line and got a yes response. It was quite detrimental to the family and therefore something that needed to be dealt with.

It can sometimes help to work out what the problem is when you know the local area well. I marked where the line ran in the house (in a north-west to south-east direction) and after firing up my computer and using a local map, extended it to see where it led.

It went straight through a boarding kennels and my eyes flicked upwards, my yes response, telling me that this was the source, now all that I had to do was find how and why it came into existence. That is how 'Animal Created Stress Lines' entered my remit.

They are very similar to the stress lines that we humans have created, but these are caused by the suffering of animals, mentally and physically. The boarding kennels have a good reputation locally and the line was not caused by cruelty, but the unhappiness, anxiety and grieving, of dogs and cats that were staying there whilst their owners were on holiday.

They were suffering from mental stress, not knowing if they had been abandoned or would ever see their owners again. The same thing happens, but to a lesser degree, if they are left alone in the house for hours whilst their owners are at work and I have found this to be the cause since discovering these lines.

I would always suggest that animal owners talk to their pet, explaining why they are being left at kennels and how long for. That you will be returning to pick them up and that you still love them. Animals do understand what you are saying to them and by explaining the reasons why they are not in their normal home will help them on a physical and mental level.

## Case Study: A house in Leyburn, North Yorkshire

I dowsed a house in Leyburn recently and picked up various animal stress lines running through it from the local livestock auction market, these were caused by the anxiety of the animals being sold. The same would be true if you lived near an abattoir, but I would expect those lines to be far more detrimental to both you and the family.

If you have an animal rescue centre nearby, you may find yourself with a full-time job clearing these stress lines because there will be similar levels of unhappiness and anxiety in the animals there, similar to the boarding kennels mentioned earlier.

If you find one or more of these stress lines, there are several ways that you can help.

First, send healing to the animals, then to those who are working with the animals, and then make sure that the kennels are clear of all detrimental emotion, other forms of geopathic stress and the anxiety that has built up over the years. Finally, send healing along the complete length of the line or lines. The healing section at the end of the book will help you with this.

## Dowsing diagnostic questions for animal created stress lines:

1. Is the house or family affected by a stress line created by an animal?
2. Is the animal a family pet?
3. Is the stress line caused by the mental or physical suffering of a pet?
4. Is it caused by the family or owner of the pet (physical or mental abuse)?
5. Has it been caused by the pet being left for hours by themselves?
6. It is due to the pet being left at a boarding kennels and pining for their owners?
7. Is it due to the lack of mental or physical stimulation of a pet/animal?
8. Is it due to the lack of attention/affection?
9. How long is the line?
10. Can it all be healed?
11. Will there be any layers to work in (days, weeks, months)?
12. Do I send healing to the individual animals or can this be done en masse?
13. Do the owners/staff at the kennels/rescue centre need to have healing as well?

49

# 50. Any beneficial areas to sit/meditate

A client once told me, 'the report that you provided us was very dark, and there is only one nice question on your checklist.'

My response?

You are asking me to find out what is affecting you and the family in detrimental ways and to clear these noxious energies from your home, thereby allowing you all to live a more healthy and peaceful life. Get rid of the bad stuff and the good can only get better.

But it's true that by searching out beneficial areas, you can further enhance and nurture them over time to improve the overall feeling of harmony and wellbeing in your home. If the house does not have one occurring naturally, they can be created by thoughtful and repeated meditation and/or intention, as well as in a room that is used for healing purposes, whether you see clients or carry out distant healing.

These areas are energetically special; if you find one naturally occurring in your home then you have hit the jackpot, if you find two or more, well, that is truly exceptional. They are perfect for healing purposes, not only for yourself but your family too.

If you are a Complementary therapist or involved in any form of healing (Reiki, homeopathy, massage, hypnotherapy) then this is the place for your clients to sit as whilst you work on them. Placing a chair or healing couch above these special areas will certainly benefit your clients and

50

enhance the healing energies available to you.

These areas are also perfect to meditate within or above. I would not necessarily suggest sleeping on or above one for any great length of time as this form of sacred energy and is more beneficial in small doses. Children would also benefit for sitting here, it would certainly help with their homework, as they would be receiving divine inspiration.

Once I have finished healing a home, everywhere in the house becomes beneficial, but these specific areas will always remain special and are to be treasured.

Whether you are healing, meditating, sitting in quiet contemplation or just want a place to chill, these spaces are perfect and wonderful to experience.

In my last three homes, each of the best 'hot spots' have been where I have my office. But the downside is that Annie, our Springer Spaniel, sensed exactly where they were located and always makes a beeline for them, beating me to it every time. Once settled she rarely moves unless I am making toast.

## Dowsing diagnostic questions for beneficial areas:

1. Are there any beneficial areas in the house?
2. How many?
3. Where is it/are they?
4. Is it/are they beneficial for the whole family?
5. Is it/are they good for sitting in for healing purposes?
6. Can I carry out healing from the area/s?
7. Is there a particularly good time to use the area/s?
8. Can I enhance the energies in the area/s?
9. How can I do this? Further meditation, etc.
10. Where is the best location for me to create a healing area?
11. How long will it take to create if I meditate there every day?
12. Once formed can it be pinned in place?
13. Will it be a beneficial area for the whole family?
14. Can the beneficial energy be felt on all the floor levels?

50

# 51. Energising/Healing Rays

It is well known that colours can heal, whether through crystals, clothing or simply seeing a rainbow, they all bring joy into your life, and joy is a great healer.

Our auras are made up of many different colours and shades, so is it therefore surprising to discover that the colours we dress ourselves in can have a beneficial as well as a detrimental effect, not just on us but also others?

Colours can attract and also repel. Wearing a red tie was often thought to show an aggressive nature, for instance. Some colours can appear masculine whilst others very feminine, the way we dress and the colours we chose can, outwardly, say a lot about us. I know that I feel very different when I wear my favourite aquamarine coloured sweatshirt than I do wearing my red fleece top, I feel softer, I guess is the best word to describe the feeling.

The effects of colour on humans have been understood and used for many different purposes over the years. Pastel shades can be calming for patients and they are often used in doctor's surgeries and hospitals. But in office buildings they would create the wrong atmosphere, you want your staff to be dynamic and energised, so vivid colours are the better choice.

The same goes for bedrooms, living rooms, kitchens and other parts of the home. Each room needs to reflect our moods or to help create one. We can influence and strengthen our auras by the colours in a room or with the clothes that we wear and also through visualisation. By bringing a missing colour to mind and then drawing it directly into your body and each layer of our aura can both energize and help us heal.

Each colour vibrates at slightly different levels and it is our reaction to these pulses of energy that will be beneficial to us. This is only my take on how I feel they can be of benefit to us. If you're not sure what colours you need, dowsing can help pick out the most suitable colour for you. Just ask 'Which colour is most beneficial for me to wear today?' whilst standing in front of your wardrobe, or have a colour chart in your hand, and see which direction your rod points in. You might be surprised.

Treat your body and aura separately, they may need the same colour, but that is not always the case. You may need to treat each of your auric fields separately, and your body too. Some fields of your aura may need an energizing colour whilst others need colours to calm them down.

First, check your body. You can dowse or use your intuition and ask if there is a colour that is missing or needs strengthening. To help find the right colour, visualise a rainbow starting from red and work your way through to purple. You can include the infrareds, but they are rarely needed.

Do ask about aquamarine, as this colour is becoming more essential to us as we move through the 21st century. It vibrates, to me, at a holy level, and is associated with the thymus chakra (upper heart chakra) that has opened up in recent years. This is our natural connection or link to Upstairs and Mother Earth.

I find this is the first time that the thymus chakra and aquamarine colour has appeared in the human body, and, to me, denotes that as a race, we are becoming more spiritual.

If your dowsing indicates that blue is missing, for instance, ask how long you need to sit quietly for (or meditate) whilst the colour fills up your aura and/or your body and can ask which of your auric fields needs the colour and why.

They are:

2. Etheric Body

3. Emotional Body

4. Mental Body

5. Astral Body

6. Etheric template

7. Celestial Body

8. Causal Body

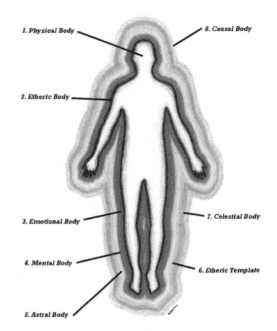

There are various ways of receiving the colours, you can wear an item of coloured clothing, picture the colour or colours wrapping around you like a shawl, or visualise it surrounding the outer perimeter of your aura and slowly drawing it towards you through each of the auric fields until it reaches your physical body. It then enters the body and fills it with the colour before finishing up centred and then absorbed by your solar plexus chakra.

You can also use crystals that correspond with your missing colour or colours, just sit and hold them in your hands and allow the vibrational energies to move through your body and then expand pushing through to the very edges of your auric field.

If I am working on a client, normally from a distance, I will arrange a specific time for them to sit quietly, preferably by themselves, I then psychically (vibrationally) transfer the specific colour or colours to them for as long as is necessary. I focus on them and in my mind's eye see them sitting on a cushion. I see that the whole of their aura is filled with the necessary colour, rather like a thick mist, swirling all around them.

Gradually it forms a solid band at the outer edges, slowly moving through each of the seven different fields, it reduces in size the closer it gets to the physical body shrinking, finally to cellular level, ending up entering the solar plexus chakra.

These are not the colours of the chakras; this is a very different way of healing. These rays replace the missing or faded colours that have been gradually eroded due to our modern lifestyle.

Weekly commuting on trains or buses allows fellow passengers to drain you of your energy (life force) unless you have fully protected yourself. Most people won't realise that this is happening, whilst others definitely will. So-called Psychic Vampires can steal your colours, so keep your guard up, and finally, when you get home, replenish your energy, checking for your faded or missing colours, then sit down quietly and top them up.

This will help you relax and aid both your mental and physical wellbeing.

## Dowsing diagnostic questions for energising/healing rays:

1. Am I missing any colours that are important to me?
2. Which ones?
3. Can they be restored?
4. Can I do this using healing?
5. How long do I need to sit and bring in the colours for?
6. Do any of the colours need strengthening?
7. Which ones?
8. How long do I need to do this healing for?
9. Would I benefit from sitting in a coloured beam?
10. Which colour or coloured beams do I need?
11. How long do I need to sit for?
12. Is there a colour that I need to wear today?
13. Will this help in the healing process?
14. Is this something that I should do daily/weekly?

51

# 52. Anything else to be considered regarding the health of the people

In this section, we are dowsing to see if there is anything else needed to improve the health of you and the family or the people whose home we are dowsing. It includes vitamins, minerals, therapies and essences.

I have nothing but praise for Bach Flower Remedies. I know that some people feel that they are out of date for use in the 21st Century, but it is sometimes good to rely on tried and tested methods and I tend to view them in different ways to many practitioners.

During a diagnosing session, I dowse to find out which particular remedy is needed for each member of the family in order to help them adjust to the changing energies in their home as the healing takes place. It helps their mind and body adapt to the new patterns coming in as the old and unwanted energies start to dissipate.

I have often heard clients say, 'You must have met my husband/wife, as that is exactly what they are like', but on some occasions the remedies that I dowsed for were almost the opposite of a person's characteristics and I admit to finding that a little disconcerting to begin with and thought that my dowsing must be wrong.

However, as I started to fine-tune the healing process, reacting to the regular feedback from my client and family, I began to realise that the remedies were exactly what was needed. By being the total opposite of their character, they were helping to bring a new balance into that

52

person's life. There is a reason for everything, and it sometimes takes you a little while to realise exactly what the reason is.

Historically, the remedies have always had a minute amount of alcohol in them acting as a preservative, but in recent years an alcohol-free remedy has been developed using glycerine as the additive. I work out how many drops my client and their individual family members will need, what time of day they should take them and for how long.

I recommend that they put the drops in a small tumbler of water (ideally filtered) and to sip it slowly. I know that some people will circumvent this and put the drops directly under their tongue, but I find it more beneficial for them to be absorbed through the stomach.

There is also another way of taking these remedies, as some of my client's family members are occasionally averse to taking anything that might be considered 'alternative', or 'Quack Medicine' as one teenage son politely put it, and that is by sending it vibrationally.

It may sound farfetched, but as you know, everything is energy and these remedies each have their own specific vibration, so why can't we send that particular frequency to the client over the airwaves?

The diagram on the next page is called an 'Energy Teleporter' and was written about in *Spirit & Earth*. It is a method of sending the healing energy of the chosen essence or remedy through the ether. You place the remedy bottle (or the name of it) on the 'Transmit' section of the diagram and the name of the recipient on 'Absorb', then walk away and let it do its stuff.

I suggest that you photocopy a number of these diagrams to save spoiling the book as you begin to use them more and more, not just for yourself or immediate family, but also for your friends. If you have a remedy that you wish to take yourself, place a glass of water on 'Absorb' and the name of the remedy of your choice on 'Project', dowse how long it needs to be there for, to fully take in the healing vibration, then once done, pick it up and sip it slowly.

52

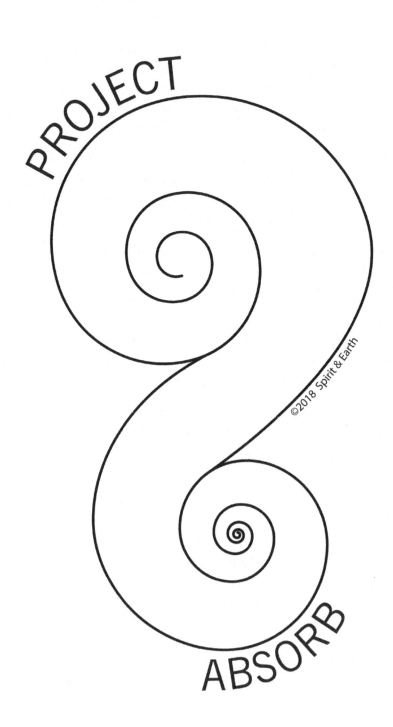

PROJECT

ABSORB

©2018 Spirit & Earth

52

You can also use the healing power of crystals and/or sacred symbols by placing them on 'PROJECT' and a glass of water on 'ABSORB', dowse the length of time needed for the process to work, and then when ready, slowly drink the water.

There are also many sacred symbols you could use; this depends on what you want them to do. There is the Flower of Life, Metatron's Cube, the Arwen, Om, the Merkaba, Vesica Pisces, Antahkarana and many more, each vibrating at a different level.

Symbols can be used for protection; and some can be invigorating whilst others will help to strengthen your mind and body. I dowse to find out if an essence is needed or whether a symbol is required and how long they need to remain on the card for maximum benefit.

Experiment to find the best solution, just ensure that the healing is the most appropriate for the person concerned and working for their highest good. That way, you cannot go wrong.

You can also dowse to see if you would benefit from a particular healing session or therapy, there are just too many to choose from for me to list.

## Dowsing diagnostic questions for treatments/therapies:

1. Would I benefit from a therapy? Which one?
2. How many weeks would I need to go?
3. Who is the best person to see?
4. Am I short of any vitamins?
5. Which ones?
6. Would a course of, say vitamin $D_3$ (or any other), benefit me?
7. How long should I take them for?
8. Which brand is best for me?
9. Am I short of minerals?
10. Which ones?
11. Would a course be of benefit?
12. How long do I/we need take them for?

52

13. Do I need a particular essence?
14. Which make is best for me at this time?
15. Which essence do I need?
16. How long do I need it for?
17. When do I need to take it? (am or pm)
18. How many drops do I need?
19. Will it help my energy levels?

# 53. Is there anything else that is detrimental for me to find?

Potentially, this is one of the most time-consuming questions to ask because if you get a yes response from your rod or pendulum you will need to work out what and where the detrimental energies are coming from also what you can do about them. You may have to work through a myriad of questions before getting the correct answer.

This very open question is the reason why I have written this book as a follow up to *Heal Your Home*. You ask the question and wait with bated breath for the pendulum to move, if it doesn't, you breathe a sigh of relief, however if you get a yes response, then the head scratching starts.

It can be quite frustrating just when you feel you have cleared and healed everything, to find there is something else to do. Once you have worked out exactly what the problem is, the exasperation turns to exhilaration. Patience and perseverance really does pay off.

I once considered my original checklist to be exhaustive, and cover every possible issue, but I have proved myself wrong. The new questions in this book have moved my healing, literally, into a different dimension.

## Case Study: Indigenous spirits

I have recently worked on a house situated on the West Coast of the USA, where I came across ancient Indigenous spirits that needed help.

The case was an interesting one as the lady concerned had many problems

279

inside the house that needed to be cleared and then healed. There was a lot of detrimental earth energies as, unbeknownst to me, the area contains a number of non-active volcanoes and over millions of years they had created a series of tubes running beneath the ground as well as leaving exposed lava flows on the surface of the earth.

These upheavals had caused the energies locally to become rather jumbled and distorted, the water had been affected too and it was certainly an interesting project to work on. There was also a recurring problem of any time she brought anything new into the house the item or items would begin to radiate detrimental energy and, in many cases, had to be thrown away.

I worked on clearing anything in the house that might be causing this to happen. Several spirits moved into the light, a life form was removed, water veins were dealt with and several energy spirals were harmonised. The owner also had problems with neighbours, one woman in particular was psychically attacking her, so healing was sent, and we saw a brief period of calm, which didn't last.

She thought that there may be a curse on the land, but I had already checked that and did not find anything that was detrimental to her. There was something showing up in the corner of her garden that wasn't quite right, but it had not yet fully appeared. This can be a problem when dealing with layers and you have to work on them one level at a time and you cannot move on to the next layer until you have successfully dealt with the current one.

This turned out to be the case. I finally began to feel that we were reaching the final stages of the healing, the last level. As we did, it turned out to be both interesting and humbling.

My client was a very sensitive lady and often felt a dark presence when she was in the garden. Her dogs did too, there was one area that they actively avoided and at its centre was a large bush. One day, she decided to cut it down and that is when the final layer made itself well and truly known, just as she was pulling out the roots. The more she cleared, the bigger the hole became; she suddenly became very aware of the dark presence and knew it had emanated from the hole.

53

I received an email informing me that she had removed the bush and what she had experienced when the presence had made itself known. I tuned in and replied 'The dark energy that you experienced is made from the emotions of others, ancient stuff – around the late 1500s into the 1600s. It is not human, but a free-floating form made up of the dark thoughts, actions, hurt, agony, suffering and upset of the local population at that time, an Indigenous tribe. I would refer to the presence as a 'Human Manifested Thought Form'.

It took a number of months to clear this energy from the tunnel, but every time it appeared to have gone it would suddenly reappear a few days later, weaker, but still there. So, I had to devise a new way of working on this thought form to fully remove it.

The hole, it seems, was a natural tunnel or tube created by an erupting volcano millions of years ago and was discovered and used by the Indigenous population as a place to go when feeling unwell, rather like an isolation ward in a hospital. But as the white settlers flooded into the area, they brought diseases like smallpox, measles and typhoid with them, infecting many of the local tribes, so the tunnel then became a place to go and die.

I decided to call on the individual spirits (they had already gone to the light), who over the years, were responsible for its creation. I asked each of them to come back down to Earth (in spirit form), to remove the individual emotion energy patterns that had combined to create this dark form. This took several hours to complete. Gradually, the energies were nibbled away at and individually taken to the light. Finally, the hurt and upset that had brought the thought form into existence had been removed.

Then there were a number of layers left to heal, firstly helping a further sixty-five Indigenous people travel to the light. Each tribe has its own conviction on the hereafter, but I do believe they share a common belief in Grandfather, The Ancient One or Great Spirit.

53

The spirits had been down in the tunnel for centuries, afraid to come out and therefore unable to visit Grandfather Sky. I tried to work out as best I could which tribe they came from, found a traditional chant and performed a short ceremony allowing them to meet their ancestors. I

281

had also called on one of my guides, Eagle That Soars, to help with the process.

**Update:** 25th January 2021.

Further problems have come to light since, what I felt, was the final clearing. Part of this dark form had not gone, even though, at the time it felt as if it had. My advice is, keep checking for layers, just in case.

In this instance I had to think outside the box as something else had to be done to clear the area of this misery, upset and death. An image came into my head of the transporter in Start Trek, giving them the ability to beam people to and from any given location, I asked if this was appropriate for what I needed to do and got an affirmative answer back.

So, in my head I imagined the dark form, and anything associated with it, being held within a beam of white light asking for them to be 'transported' into the Universe. This seemingly took place and automatically I became aware of a further 25 lost souls, that had been held back from going to the light by this dark energy. I then performed a short ceremony helping them move through.

I finished by flooding the tunnels and surrounding area with a healing light asking that it all be left in peace balance and harmony. The final healing I performed was to lift a curse on the land, which felt like the final layer that had now come to light.

So, as you can see, by asking the question it can lead you down many pathways.

## Dowsing diagnostic questions for anything else that is detrimental to find:

1. Is there anything else that is detrimental to the family that I need to find?

2. Is it connected to any other question in the checklist?

3. Is it something from the past or present?

4. Is it caused by another human being?

5. Is it connected to an individual member of the family?

6. Have they done something to cause this problem?

7. When (try and get a date, including the month and year)?

8. Is it part of a layer system that I have not dealt with?

9. Is it above ground or below?

10. Are there lost souls attached to the problem?

11. Is it earth energies related?

12. Water related?

13. Is it linked to a neighbour?

14. Is it linked to work?

53

# 54. Family DNA clearing and healing

Deoxyribonucleic acid (DNA) is a molecule comprising two polynucleotide chains, which coil around each other forming a double helix. This carries all the instructions we need for our development, how we function, our growth and reproduction. This applies to all known organisms.

DNA is the cornerstone of life, a blueprint that encompasses complex genetic coding making us who we are, why we are and what we are.

Our DNA (double helix) is exclusive, there are no two people the same, though there is one slight exception to that rule. Identical twins came from the same initial cell and will therefore have the same DNA. I find that mind blowing because it means that every single person currently living on Earth, and all those who have ever lived before us, are 100% unique.

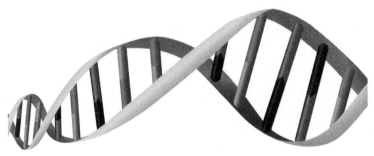

*The DNA double helix*

Then we have junk DNA, cast aside by scientists mainly because they do not know what purpose it serves in our body. It is now being referred to as non-coding. It seems they are starting to hedge their bets, just in case.

I believe that everything in our body has a function, and a reason for being there, it does not matter how small or insignificant it is. Cells, for instance, are microscopic, but each has its purpose.

So, all of who we are is down to genetic coding; that includes your sex, the colour of your eyes, your height, your stature, skin tone etc. All of this has come down the family line, from every one of your ancestors, the good and bad.

Wouldn't it be amazing if we could send healing back through the ages, to our earliest ancestor, to correct any underlying defects that have come through the family line or clear any cellular memories of an illness that has had an impact on us and our family today?

And if you begin to tune in and discover that we are, indeed, living 'Simultaneous or Parallel Lives' it makes this healing so much more precious as it can have a direct effect not only on us today but on every other life we are living. That goes for our family too.

Well, Upstairs says that we can, so who am I to argue?

This question was added to my checklist in summer 2020, and I am slowly coming to terms with the enormity of what we, as humans, can achieve if we put our minds to it.

I have no case studies as yet, but I wanted to include this information in the book so that you, the reader, can start to expand the range of your healing to include all of your ancestors, but before you do so, make sure that they have all gone to the light. You may be surprised to find that one or two may be still hanging around but are now ready to go.

I would like to think that we can send healing back along our family line, to the earliest of our ancestors, clearing away all the hardship, emotional stress, hunger, physical and mental pain, death, or trauma.

54

If we do so, I feel that it could make such a difference to our lives today, because part of the healing process would include clearing away any cellular memory of inherited diseases including Malaria, typhoid, smallpox, syphilis and gonorrhoea, tuberculosis, leprosy, pneumonia, or polio.

I have compiled a list of questions to help you determine whether or not there is any point to this healing and if, as you do so, whether it will make any difference to you and your family's health today.

Please do send me any thoughts you may have, or any insights once you have carried out a healing.

## Dowsing diagnostic questions for family DNA clearing and healing:

1. Is it possible for me to clear and heal my DNA?
2. If it is, how far, or how many generations, do I need to go back?
3. Is there anything in particular that needs to be cleared or healed?
4. Will this help me and future generations?
5. How detrimentally am I or members of my family affected by these mutated cells? (scale of 0 to -10)
6. Is it possible for me to clear and heal any detrimental cellular memory that is affecting me?
7. Or any members of my family?
8. Again, how far back to I need to go?
9. How beneficial will this be? Use scale of 0 to +10.
10. Are there many layers to heal? Both DNA and Cellular memory.
11. Is the cellular memory of a particular illness or disease?
12. Does it come through my Maternal or Paternal line?
13. Will this heal my DNA in my parallel and simultaneous lives?

54

# Part Four

*Healing*

# Preparing to Heal

Before you begin to heal your home, you must ensure you are fully psychically protected. So, if you have not yet done so, please take the time now to go through the psychic protection method.

It is essential that this protection process becomes part of your daily ritual, and I cannot emphasise or stress this enough. When you are carrying out any form of healing, psychic protection is of paramount importance. And even when you are not, it is essential for your own daily wellbeing and that of your family.

Detrimental energy patterns are all around us, whether they come from earth energies or people's emotional outpourings, so if you are a sensitive and open person then you stand a good chance of picking up something nasty.

A lot of therapists and healers call me for help, having picked up an attachment or worse after giving healing to a client. Often, when someone is receiving healing they start to relax and begin to release their pent-up emotions, all that anxiety, worry, stress, trauma and fear has to go somewhere, and the healer is directly in the firing line.

A huge tidal wave of guilt and long buried memories can also be released, some of them will be absorbed into the fabric of the room (not good if you work from home), and also the healing couch. Worse still is when they become attached to the healer, repeatedly.

'Spiritual Hygiene' is the key to remaining clear of these detrimental energies.

All healers should protect themselves before they see a client, and ideally, carry out a clearing on the client before they come into the healing room. Then, once the session is finished, ensure that anything detrimental left behind by the client is also cleared away so that it will not have an ill effect on the therapist or their next client.

The same goes for all therapy work, massages, homeopathy, hypnotherapy, hairdressers, and anyone, in fact, who gets close to another human being and/or has any form of physical contact.

Anyone moving through your auric fields can pose a threat. Imagine you are standing on a crowded underground train; how many people are you interacting with? Fifteen or twenty, perhaps more? Your aura can extend some 25ft, sometimes further, and of course so does everyone else's. Subconsciously, you will be picking up a lot of information from almost every person in the carriage and much of it will not be very healthy.

Anything that was attached to them can now easily move across to merging into any of your auric fields. That sudden headache is a tell-tale sign, as is a sudden drop in energy or the onset of nausea or dizziness. The same thing can happen to your children when attending school, so it is never too early to sit them down and explain how they can surround themselves with beautiful rainbow colours. It's a fun spiritual hygiene practice that will keep them safe and free from attachments and other people's emotional junk. You never know, they might be able to see and/ or feel the colours moving into and out of their body, they just hadn't mentioned it before because to them it is normal.

## Psychic Protection Method:

I would suggest that you carry out this exercise each morning and especially before you start to do any healing work on other people and/ or your home. It is essential that you are clear of any 'nasties' before you do any healing work, this helps you become a clear channel for the light.

Any attachments would mean that a) you might pass them on to others and b) your healing will not be as affective.

We use the solar plexus chakra as our centre point. Each colour we breathe in gathers there, at cellular level, and on the out breath it expands, moving through our physical body, cleansing it of everything detrimental to us. It then continues to the outer edge of our auric field, cleansing that too. Each colour then shrinks, to create bands of protection around our body.

Don't forget, that apart from the crown and base chakras, we have chakras at the back of our body too. Therefore when breathing in do include the colours entering from the back.

Before we start, we need to read the following and ask that this happens each time we breathe out the specified colour, you only need to set the intention once, not on each breath:

**'I ask that, as I breathe out, my body (at cellular level) and aura are cleared of all detrimental and inappropriate attachments, all lower animal life forms, their seeds and tentacles, all human manifested thought forms and life forms, all worries and concerns, any miasms and detrimental family DNA, any cancers and tumours, any past, present and parallel life traumas or upsets, all detrimental parental patterning, all parasites and any other detrimental energies that are inappropriate to me. I also request that all unnecessary psychic and physical cords are cut and everything that has been removed or dislodged be taken to the light and disposed of appropriately. I ask that the healing takes place not only in this dimension but all other dimensions that are similarly affected.'**

Once you have made the above request, either silently or out loud, sit quietly and take two deep breaths.

First, visualise breathing in the colour **brown** through the chakras found on the soles of your feet. See this moving up your legs to your solar plexus, then forming a glowing ball of light at cellular level. As you breathe out, visualise it expanding through your body and outwards to the outer edge of your auric field, cleansing the body and aura of all detrimental and inappropriate energy patterns. It then shrinks to form a two-inch layer of brown around your physical body, this is your connection to Mother Earth.

Then breathe in **red ochre (reddish brown)** through the chakras found in each knee. Bring this up to your solar plexus through your legs, and your body via your base/root chakra and pranic tube. From here, see it expanding through your body to the outer edge of your aura, cleansing the body and aura of all detrimental energy patterns. It then shrinks to form a two-inch layer of reddish brown around your physical body, over the brown protective barrier.

Next breathe in **red**, through your base chakra up to your solar plexus via your pranic tube. At the top of your breath, exhale. Expand this healing colour through your body to the edge of your aura, cleansing both of all detrimental energy patterns and then it shrinks to form a third layer around you, over the red ochre barrier.

Next breathe in **orange**, through the front and back of your sacral chakra up to your solar plexus via your pranic tube. At the top of your breath, exhale. Expand this healing colour through your body to the edge of your aura, cleansing both of all detrimental energy patterns and then it shrinks to form a fourth layer around you, over the red.

Next breathe in **yellow**, through the front and back of your solar plexus chakra. At the top of your breath, exhale, pushing the healing light through your body to the outer edge of your aura. This cleans all detrimental energy patterns, shrinking to form a fifth layer around you, over the orange layer, just like the layers of an onion.

Breathe **green** in through the front and back of your heart chakra, and down into your solar plexus via your pranic tube. As you exhale, push the colour through your body to the outer edge of your auric field, cleansing the body and aura. It then shrinks, to form a sixth layer around you.

Breathe **aquamarine** into the front and back of your thymus (or upper heart) chakra and feel it moving down to your solar plexus. Exhale and push the colour through your body to the outer edge of your auric field – cleansing it. Then allow it to shrink to form the seventh layer around you.

Breathe in **light blue** through the front and back of your throat chakra down into your solar plexus via your pranic tube. Exhale to push the colour through your body and aura, then shrink it to form the eighth layer.

Breathe **dark blue** in through the front and back of your third eye/brow chakra down into your solar plexus via your pranic tube. Exhale to push the colour through your body and aura, then shrink to form a ninth layer.

Through your crown chakra, breathe in **purple** sending it down to your solar plexus. Exhale to cleanse the body and aura, then see it shrink to become the tenth protective layer.

Then breathe in a **silver** light through your crown chakra, into your solar plexus. Exhale, and push it through your body and aura. It shrinks to form the eleventh layer.

Breathe in a **gold** light, via your crown chakra, down to your solar plexus and as you exhale push it through your body and aura, cleansing them of all detrimental energy patterns. It shrinks to form the twelfth and final protective barrier.

Finally breathe in **divine white light**, via your crown chakra, see it filling up your body from the tips of your toes to the top of your head.

You are now fully protected; your chakras are cleansed, as is your body and auric field.

Please, please, please get into the habit of doing this exercise daily, ideally before you get out of bed in the morning. Use the quiet few minutes after you wake up to clear and protect yourself. You should only need to do this once a day but check that the protection is still in place before embarking on any healing work. The more you practice, the quicker you will get until it fits perfectly into your regular breathing pattern. It can also be carried out whilst in the shower, but please do not try whilst driving as the temptation will be there for you to close your eyes to visualise the colours.

# How to carry out a healing safely

Once you have fully protected yourself, the next thing to ensure, before you begin the healing part of the process, is that you are not using your own energy to do so. If you do, you are asking for trouble, maybe not in the short term but certainly in the medium to long term. If you keep doing so your internal batteries are going to be depleted and you will start to suffer from many different aches and pains, lack of energy, brain fog etc., and eventually will suffer from a spiritual burn out.

Many healers have suffered early deaths, due to their life force having been drained away. They had freely given healing to others, but this was using their core 'inner' energy. Once it ran out there was no going back.

Therefore, we need to find an external source or sources that have a limitless supply of energy that we can channel to help ourselves and to send to others. Welcome to Upstairs, the Management, The Powers that Be, the Highest of the High, God, the Universe, Jehovah, Allah or simply The Light. Feel free to call this higher power whatever you feel comfortable with or what your belief codes dictate.

You need to learn how to **CHANNEL** this vital energy, a boundless source of healing light, allowing it to safely enter your body, sending it out to whomever you are working on. Whether they are sitting right in front of you or living a thousand miles away, the effect will still be the same.

To do this we need to 'tune in', to make it known to the higher power that we wish to connect with them and start to absorb, then channel the healing white light.

## How do we tune in?

With reverence and great respect.

I liken tuning in to opening the office door in the morning and getting yourself ready for the day. It opens you up and changes (elevates) your vibrational energy, and you become an available vessel that Spirit will then use to send healing. You can dictate when this happens (as you have free will) and switch it off when you feel that you have had enough, thereby returning yourself and the energy of your body to 'normal living levels'. This is essential for your wellbeing.

Performing any form of healing can be exhausting, especially when you first start. Channelling the light from Spirit can be exhilarating but can leave you feeling exhausted. The more experience you have, the better you become at handling these heavenly energies. But even with experience you will find that most humans are incapable of staying in this higher vibrational state for any length of time, therefore it is important to close down at the end of each session returning to a 'physical' grounded way of life.

I always light a candle before I start and then recite The Lord's Prayer. The words are so ingrained after years of reciting them during school assemblies that it seems to be a natural way to begin a healing session, but I have made a number of changes to reflect the beings that I now connect with:

**Our Father who art in Heaven,**

**Our Mother who is on Earth,**

**Our Life-Giving Sun and Heavenly Moon hallowed be thy names.**

**Thy Kingdom come**

**Thy will be done on earth, as it is in heaven**

**Give us this day our daily bread**

**And forgive us our trespasses,**

As we forgive those that trespass against us
And lead us not into temptation
But deliver us from evil
For thine is the kingdom
The power, and the glory
For ever and ever
Amen.

I know that some people don't like the wording, and that there are a number of modern-day variations flying about, but I still like the one that I grew up with (with my additions). The choice is yours, whatever you feel comfortable reciting, it is not just the words but the intention behind the words. Your way of mentally leaving the physical world behind and connecting to the spiritual.

I will often have music playing quietly in the background. I love Karunesh especially and find that most of his music feels very right for what I am doing.

Once I have tuned in, I then ask the following:

**'To the Highest of the High, Mother Earth, Our Life Giving Sun and Heavenly Moon, please hear my prayer and in doing so allow me to connect to the power of the Universe, to use that energy in my healing. I ask that I am a clear healing channel and my healing be of the highest standard and working for the higher good of all the people and animals that come into my conscious and subconscious mind during the day. And to enlist the help from the following:**

**Master Jesus**
**Akhenaten**
**Saint Germain**
**The Maitreya Buddha and the psychic and healing energies coming from Arcturus and Maldek.'**

(Arcturus is a powerful psychic star system and Maldek was a planet situated between Mars and Jupiter, its remains are what is called the Asteroid Belt. It was destroyed millennia ago by ego but still transmits some powerful energies.)

The following Archangels:

Metatron

Michael

Sammuel

Azriel

Feriel

Uriel

Zadkiel

Geburatiel

All other Archangels and Angels that need to be with me today

All appropriate spirits

My Spirit Guides

My Protection Guides

My Healing Guides

The Goddess Sateri (a recent addition to my spiritual team)

Hatshepsut (the Egyptian Pharaoh)

Eagle that Soars (an Indian Shaman and Chief that I helped move to the light)

Si (my Chinese sage and Master Healer)

Arwena (a very protective female Pagan warrior)

My Soul Brother (Bankinks)

John Benedict (my late Palmist friend and mentor)

Hamish Miller (late friend and earth energy dowser)

Then I am ready to start with my healing sessions.

Now, just be aware that your guides can change as can the Archangels you work with. I am happy for you to dowse my list to see if any of the above are pertinent for you to call on, otherwise do some research on the internet. Each Archangel and angel radiate colour (Michael comes in on the blue rays, Gabriel on white and Uriel via red rays for instance), you can therefore either start with a particular colour that you see or dowse for their names as you work down the list.

# Healing Methods

I would now like to describe four methods of healing that will be referred to at various times during the healing section of the book.

## The Ultra-Fine Mesh Net of Light and Love:

I liken this to a net that is pulled behind a trawler (fishing boat) but rather than picking up fish it is clearing away a lot of the emotional debris left in your home. It will also work on many other things too.

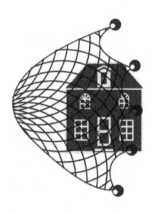 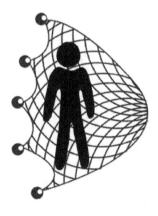

This is a good catch all, and it can be a quick fix when and if you need one. But I would always suggest that later, when you have a little more time, you double check to make sure that the problem has been cleared and that no more in-depth healing is required.

Though I always recommend a more thorough healing and working out the particulars of an issue before clearing or healing it, there are times when a quick fix is needed. Let's say that you have gone to a friend's house for a meal and suddenly you become aware that all is not well, whether you sense a detrimental presence, or your hosts don't seem their normal selves. In which case, you may need to excuse yourself and then carry out a quick healing.

I tend to find that the bathroom is the best place to go, it's quiet and no one will bother you. Allyson has got quite used to me disappearing when we are in a pub, café, or restaurant. These public spaces can be the worst places to be as they are generally a dumping ground for people's emotions.

Just be sure to ask that all parts of the issue are contained within the net, for example, seeds and tentacles if dealing with lower animal life forms, and all the residue from any lost souls.

If a quick fix is needed for a specific person or home, you can recite the passages below. But as you work through each section that needs healing, you will see that we tackle one or two of these issues at a time. By doing it slowly, you are more likely to catch everything. But if time is of the essence and you are not able to pin down the specific issues, you can use this.

With this healing method, I visualise the person standing in front of the net as it is being pulled through their aura and physical body, and I recite the following (this can be out loud or in your head):

**'I ask that, as I pull the ultra-fine mesh net of light and love through (name) auric field and physical body that they are cleared of all detrimental and inappropriate attachments, all lower animal life forms their seeds and tentacles, all human manifested thought forms and life forms, cutting all psychic and physical cords that are no longer necessary, all worries and concerns, any miasms and detrimental family DNA, any cancers and tumours, any past, present, parallel and simultaneous life traumas or upsets, all detrimental parental patterning, all parasites and any other detrimental energies that are inappropriate to them. I also ask that everything that has been removed or dislodged is taken into the light and disposed of**

298

appropriately. I ask that the healing takes place not only in this dimension but all other dimensions that are similarly affected.'

If I am using this on a house, I recite the following, normally in my head:

'I ask that as the ultra-fine mesh net of light and love is being pulled through the house (above the house, below the ground and to either side as appropriate) it picks up all the energy patterns that may be affecting the family detrimentally, especially any stuck or past emotional energy areas, all detrimental bed patterns and any human manifested thought forms and life forms. I ask that the net is taken to the light and disposed of appropriately, leaving the house in peace, balance, and harmony for the family. I ask that the healing takes place not only in this dimension but all other dimensions that are similarly affected.'

This can be used anywhere, but again I would add a word of caution.

Always double check to make sure that there is nothing else that needs to be done to fully resolve the dilemma, there may be an underlying problem that needs further investigation. There could be another layer to clear, a spirit that needs help, or one or two earth energy problems that need to be dealt with.

Spirit likes you to do a good and thorough job, but they do realise that if someone needs help and we haven't the time to carry out a deep healing, using the above method is quite acceptable. But do not take liberties, you are required to put in some hard work too.

## The Spiritual Wall:

I tend to use this when I am working on a client and their family, as you can set up several spiritual waiting rooms, one for each person or member of the family, and you can include pets. This allows you to carry out a general clearing on them all, at the same time.

The idea is for each member of the family (and pets if required) to have their own spiritual waiting room. If you wish, you can visualise them sitting quietly on a chair until they are ready to stand up and move through the spiritual wall.

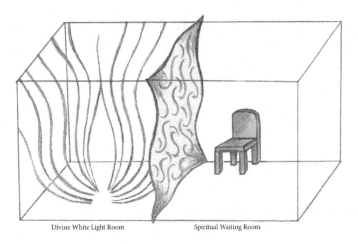

Divine White Light Room       Spiritual Waiting Room

The spiritual wall is not solid, but is made up of millions of microscopic holes, they are so small that anything detrimental or inappropriate (such as attachments) cannot pass through and are left behind as the person or pet moves from one room to another.

As they stand up and walk towards the spiritual wall, their auric field moves through first, followed by their physical body, and as this happens, I recite the following:

**'To the Highest of the High as (name or names) walks through the spiritual wall I ask that their auric fields and physical body are cleared of all detrimental and inappropriate attachments, all lower animal life forms their seeds and tentacles, all human manifested thought forms and life forms, all detrimental psychic and physical cords to be cut, clearing all worries and concerns, any miasms and detrimental family DNA, any cancers and tumours, any past, present, parallel and simultaneous life traumas or upsets, all detrimental parental patterning, all parasites and any other detrimental energies that are inappropriate to them at this stage. I ask that the healing takes place not only in this dimension but all other dimensions that are similarly affected.'**

I then ask for **'Anything that has been removed, dislodged or left behind in the spiritual waiting room is to be taken to the light and disposed of appropriately.'**

Once they have walked through the wall and completely moved into the divine white light room, I provide them with full protection, either

300

surrounding them with the multitude of colours as per my psychic protection method, or by placing them in a bubble of white light and placing mirrors on the outside to reflect anything detrimental coming towards them. The person or persons will stay in the divine white light room for as long as their higher self deems necessary, when the healing has reached its conclusion, they will naturally leave the room. (You don't have to consciously move them from the room).

## Connecting with the Natural Energies to remove detrimental attachments

Wherever possible, I like to use the natural energies that surround us to assist with healing, and these include the healing light from Spirit, the energies of Mother Earth, the life-giving qualities of our Sun and the heavenly beauty of the moon. We would not be here if it were not for the combination of all four.

I normally carry out this exercise once a week on myself, Allyson and Annie (the Springer), ensuring that we are all clear and that nothing nasty has attached itself to us. Just to reiterate an earlier comment, Spiritual Hygiene is so important, and it should feature regularly in your life, whether you are involved in carrying out holistic therapies or not.

I will also use this 'Natural Connection' method frequently when working on clients; it really is a toss-up as to whether I work this way or use the Spiritual Wall method. They are both as effective as each other, I will leave you to choose which one you prefer.

You can also carry out this exercise remotely, picturing the person or family member in your mind (a photograph might help you to concentrate on them) as you do the following:

**Step 1:** Sit quietly for a few minutes, with both feet firmly on the floor, listen to your breathing and feel the coolness of air entering your body and the warmth as you exhale. Do this for a few minutes until you feel nice and relaxed.

**Step 2:** Imagine roots growing out of your feet into Mother Earth, (it doesn't matter if you cannot visualise it, just ask for it to happen), they penetrate deeper and deeper into the planet until they reach the centre.

The whole core is an aquamarine crystal (or a crystal of your choice) and the roots wrap themselves around it grounding you and fully connecting you to the Earth.

A healing light (the colour of your chosen crystal) will naturally begin to rise, entering your body via your feet (you may suddenly feel warmer or experience a tingling sensation) and travel up your legs passing through your base and sacral chakras and into your solar plexus. It is then held there as a minute ball of light (as small as one of your cells).

**Step 3:** Begin to connect with Upstairs; by asking for (or visualising) a beam of healing white light, from the Source, to enter your crown chakra, which then travels down through your third eye, throat, thymus (sometimes called the upper heart) and heart chakras finally entering your solar plexus chakra where it blends with the healing ball of light from Mother Earth.,

**Step 4:** Then ask for the healing energy (power) of the sun to enter your body. This is via the front and back of your solar plexus chakra, as it enters, it fuses with the healing light from Spirit and Mother Earth, again at cellular level.

**Step 5:** Finally, you link into the heavenly light of our moon, visualising its beautiful bright light coating the outer edge of your aura, it then starts to shrink finally entering your body via the solar plexus chakra combining its healing energy with the ball of light already being held there.

**Step 6:** Then, starting from cellular level, visualise the ball of healing light expanding, moving outward from your solar plexus through your body and out to the extreme edge of your auric fields reciting the following:

**'As this coloured light moves through my body, from cellular level, I ask that my physical body and auric fields are cleared of all detrimental and inappropriate attachments, all lower animal life forms their seeds and tentacles, all human manifested thought forms and life forms, all detrimental psychic and physical cords to be cut, clearing all worries and concerns, any miasms and detrimental family DNA, any cancers and tumours, any past, present, parallel and simultaneous life traumas or upsets, all detrimental parental**

patterning, all parasites and any other detrimental energies that are inappropriate to them at this stage. I ask that the healing takes place not only in this dimension but all other dimensions that are similarly affected.'

**Step 7:** Then ask, **'Anything that has been removed or dislodged is now taken to the light and disposed of in an appropriate fashion.'**

## The Mirrored Pyramid:

I tend to use this method to defend a client against a heavy or prolonged period of psychic attack. It is similar to placing them in a bubble of white light with mirrors on the outside, reflecting any further inappropriate energy patterns reaching them, but I like using pyramids, there is something very mystical and solid about them. I always ask for those energies to be returned to the person responsible for sending them but send the energies with unconditional love.

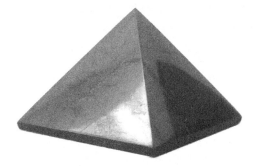

*The Mirrored Pyramid*

I always carry out a healing on the person before I place them inside the pyramid, they may have been subjected to a debilitating psychic attack or perhaps some off-world interference, so clearing those energies patterns away first is paramount.

Once they are clear, I visualise the person (family member or yourself) laying on a comfortable bed or sitting in a chair at the centre of the pyramid, and although they cannot be seen from outside, they will still be able to see people walking past, rather like a two-way mirror. So that they don't feel isolated but have 100% protection.

## Healing Protocols:

Those of you who have read *Heal Your Home* will notice that the order of the list has changed. As new questions have come through, it became important to rearrange the checklist in a more logical order.

It is helpful for you to have worked through all the questions contained in my first book, this not only shows respect to Spirit but also helps you to carry out the healing especially when it comes to helping lost souls move to the light.

## How to start:

By now, you will have worked through the checklist, and diagnosed your home. You may have already moved some spirits to the light or removed attachments from your aura, but otherwise, you will now be working on healing the home and those who reside within of anything detrimental.

Please note that I have repeated, at each stage, for you to check that your protection is in place. If you are carrying out a complete healing, then you do not have to check every time you move on to a new section. Only check if you are carrying out the healing in stages

# Dimensional Healing

I have worked on many hundreds of houses over the years, probably over a thousand, and a question that I ponder on sometimes is 'How soon after I start my work does the client and family feel the benefit of the healing?'.

Sometimes it can be immediate, almost to the second that I start to concentrate on them and sometimes it can take several days. What confounds me is when they feel the healing take place half an hour before I start my work, or a week or so later.

I received a download at the beginning of 2021 from Upstairs telling me to include the following information in this book, I hope that is goes some way to explain how to make any form of healing more effective. I have also had to change some of the wording in my invocations to take this upgrade into account.

In essence we have to send healing not only to the family living in this dimension but to those living in every other dimension that may be affected, but only as appropriate.

Why 'as appropriate'?

Because nothing should be forced. Upstairs know what they are doing, let them decide what healing is relevant. Saying that, it is good to draw their attention to these other dimensions. If you do not, they will not be included in your healing.

We need the house and family healing to take place not only in this dimension but all other dimensions that are similarly affected, in a detrimental way.

I know this paints an incredibly complex picture, and the concept can be difficult for us to grasp, but I hope that some of this was explained in the chapters on simultaneous and parallel lives. We need to expand our minds when carrying out any healing to include all aspects of our lives, those we see and feel part of, and those that we do not.

I feel that the further we move into the 21st century the more we will begin to connect with these dimensional lives, and we will become more aware as to how our actions in this life affect them, and alternatively, how their actions affect us.

We need to have an awareness of these 'other lives', and we do not necessarily need to understand how the Universe works to do so. It is simply enough to recognise that these other dimensions exist and to regularly send healing to them, especially when working on your home and family.

Sending healing to these other dimensions is rather like dropping a pebble into a still pond, and watching the ripples move outwards in ever-increasing circles. In this case you are the epicentre, and the healing focussed on you will spread outwards to all the other affected dimensions. And as with the ripples in the pond once it reaches the outer edge it will 'bounce back' moving towards the centre.

This is why healing can reach a client before I physically start my work in this dimension, because before I drop the proverbial pebble into the water, I am subconsciously thinking about doing so. This thought is the pebble, the ripples have begun.

The subconscious is therefore responsible for sending out the initial burst of healing before the conscious mind starts to focus on the task ahead. Our subconscious mind may turn out to be our natural link to the Universe. We do not fully understand how it operates but it is one of the most remarkable tools that we humans have been given.

As you work through this healing section, I'd like you to consider this quote by Dr Rodney McKay, the lead scientist of the Atlantis Expedition in the TV series Stargate Atlantis:

*'Every possible outcome to every decision ever made, exists in this multi-layer universe'.*

# Heal your Home Checklist

## Spirits, Attachments, Human Manifested Energy Forms

1.      Spirits, Ghosts, Tricky Spirits, Trapped Souls

1a.     Spirits Attached to the Auric Field

2.      Detrimental/Inappropriate Attachments

3.      Detrimental Energy Forms (Human Manifested)

4.      Lower Animal Life Forms

5.      Sorcery/Black Magic

6.      Spirit Lines

## Earth Energies

7.      Water Veins/Underground Streams

8.      Any other detrimental water source

9.      Earth Energy Lines

10.     Energy Channels

11.     Fault Lines

12.     Dynamic Energy Lines

13.     Human Intent Lines

14.     Energy Spirals

15.     Energetic Sink Holes

16.     Reversal Points

# Detrimental Human Energy Patterns

17.     Emotional Energy Areas (Human Conflict)

18.     Psychic Cords

19.     Dimensional Portals

20.     Illness Trigger Points

21.     Consecrated Ground

22.     Curses or Spells

23.     Psychic Attack

24.     Power Artefacts

25.     Place Memory

26.     Interdimensional Place Memory

27.     Vows or Contracts

28.     Fractured/Torn Souls

29.     Stress/Disturbance Lines (Man-made)

30.     Karmic Problems – Simultaneous Life Trauma

30a.    Karmic Problems – Parallel Life Trauma

31.     Detrimental Implants

32.     Toxic Lines

33.     Chakra Alignments and/or Blockages

34.     Anything else affecting the house and family (in garden/ grounds or close by)

35.     Fabric of the Building

36.     Anaesthetic Traces, Inoculations, Vaccinations, Heavy Metals

37.     Parasites

## Off-World Energies

## Technopathic Stress, Fracking

## Guardian Spirits, Elementals

## Detrimental Animal Energies

## Associated Healing

# 1. Spirits, Ghosts, Tricky Spirits, Trapped Souls

With your psychic protection shield in place, follow these steps to help move any spirits into the light that you have found in your home and surrounding neighbourhood.

**Step 1:** If the spirits have any attachments and cords carry out the following and state out loud (or in your head):

## Soul Rescue/Spirit Release Invocation:

**'I ask for an 'Ultra-Fine Mesh Net of Light and Love' to be pulled through the auras of all spirits here, to remove any attachments and cut any psychic and physical cords, either leading to them or from them, that held them back from taking their original journey into the light. Please take the net into the light and dispose of it in an appropriate fashion. Please do this for any other lost souls there may be in the local area and in any other dimensions.'**

**Step 2:** Dowse to see that all the attachments have been removed and all the appropriate cords cut, if they have not, repeat the above. If they have, continue with the following:

**'Highest of the High, please shine a beam of beautiful light in front of each lost soul and show each of them a vision of what awaits them, in Heaven. Their own idea of perfection.'**

**Step 3:** Then ask to speak directly with the spirit or spirits, saying the following spirit release invocation out loud (or in your head):

**'Ladies and gentlemen, please do not be afraid by this direct form of communication as I have been granted special dispensation to talk to you today, to help you to continue your interrupted journey into the light.**

**An 'Ultra-Fine Mesh Net of Light and Love' has been pulled through your auric fields removing any attachments and cutting any cords, leading to you or from you, that held you back, so you can now go when you are ready.**

**You have been shown a vision of what awaits you, it is perfection, a true paradise, certainly far better than staying here on this cold grey mundane earth plane. It is a beautiful place to be, and there are many people waiting for you to arrive with open arms and unconditional love.**

**Should you wish anyone from your past to be with you now, to hold your hand or just help guide you on your journey, call their name and they will appear beside you.**

**There will be no retribution for anything that you have done whilst on this earth plane, or that has been done to you, as this has been part of your life's plan. This will be explained to you, once you arrive.**

**I therefore invite you now to move into the light, and to be with your family, friends, loved ones, comrades, colleagues and pets once again.**

**Amen'**

Should there be a number of lost souls to move through this can create a herd mentality. As they start to go to the light excitement builds and a lot of energy is created, attracting other spirits that will also move through en masse. Once you have carried out the soul rescue it is fun to dowse to see how many spirits actually went to the light, you might be surprised at the number you have just helped.

**Step 4:** After waiting a few minutes, dowse to see if all the souls present have gone to the light. Then enquire if there are any others that might want and need to go to the light today. Remember the layer system; it might be that the lead spirit has now gone, freeing up other trapped souls to move through. Check for a third time, to be on the safe side – do you need to move any further spirits through?

**Step 5:** As a matter of respect, I like to ask the following:

**'To the Highest of the High, please send my love to all the souls who have just been moved into the light, ensuring they are happy there.'**

**Step 6:** Once you have worked through the above it is good to complete your task by stating the following:

**'I ask that any and all doorways opened expectedly or unexpectedly during the course of my soul rescue work are now firmly closed, and that any residue left behind is now removed and taken into the light, leaving the house in peace, balance and harmony. I ask that this takes place not only in this dimension but all other dimensions that have been affected, as appropriate.'**

The reason that you close the doors after a spirit release, is because spirits, as they move through can leave an energy trail behind them. So, by closing the doors instantly and clearing away any traces of their passing, other lost souls will not be attracted to the area.

# 1a. Spirits Attached to the Auric Field

**Step 1:** Check that it is appropriate to remove these lost souls at this time. Sometimes, they are needed by the individual and removing them could cause a lot of anxiety. It is rare that they should need to be there or stay attached, but please do check.

**Step 2:** I tend to use the Spiritual Wall method for this exercise. See the affected person sitting in the waiting room and when they are ready (or yourself if affected) walk them through the wall entering the room of divine white light, stating the following out loud:

**'As (name or names) walks through the spiritual wall into the divine white light room, I ask that their auric fields and physical body are cleared of all attached detrimental spirits and that those spirits remain in the waiting room until they are moved into the light.'**

**Step 3:** Dowse to make sure that the people affected are now completely clear of all spirits in their auric fields. If not, and this is a very rare occurrence, you will need to find out why. It may be that the spirit has attachments that need to be cleared before they can move to the light. Or they have formed a symbiotic relationship with the affected person and they still need one another for a particular reason. If that is the case, dowse to find out how long this partnership needs to last and when they can be parted, making a note on your calendar.

**Step 4:** If there are attachments, use the ultra-fine mesh net to clear them

314

and cut any cords leading to or from them, then ask for them to move into the light.

**Step 5:** Ask the question to make sure that they have gone, if not, go back and use the Soul Rescue or Spirit Release invocation, asking for the assistance from the Highest of the High.

**Step 6:** Once everything is clear, state out loud:

**'I ask that any and all doorways opened expectedly or unexpectedly during the course of my soul rescue work are now firmly closed, and that any residue left behind is now removed and taken into the light, leaving the house in peace, balance and harmony.'**

# 2. Detrimental/Inappropriate Attachments

We are going to use the Ultra-Fine Mesh Net of Light and Love method to remove these little nasties from within your aura and physical body also of your family members. And, if you found any lower animal life forms in your questioning, you can now clear them at the same time with the following process.

**Step 1:** With your psychic protection in place, repeat the following invocation either out loud or in your head:

**'To the Highest of the High I ask that, as I pull the ultra-fine mesh net of light and love through (name/s) auric field and physical body that they are cleared of all detrimental and inappropriate attachments, and all lower animal life forms, including their seeds and tentacles. I also ask that everything that has been removed or dislodged is taken into the light and disposed of appropriately. I ask that the healing takes place not only in this dimension but all other dimensions that are similarly affected.'**

**Step 2:** Dowse to check that you and your family members are now completely clear of all detrimental attachments in their auras and physical body.

**Step 3:** If they are not clear, then I would suggest that you switch to using the *'Connecting with the Natural Energies'* method as it works in a slightly different way and may be more appropriate. Once done check

316

again to make sure that everyone is clear.

**Step 4:** Do ensure that your psychic protection is still in place, make sure that this is something that you do every day, it will ensure that you are kept free of any detrimental energies that may attach to you.

2

# 3. Detrimental Energy Forms (Human Manifested)

**Step 1:** Dowse to check your psychic protection is in place

**Step 2:** Visualise all of the life forms and thoughts forms (although you would be unlucky to find more than one or two in your home) being gathered together and then say either out loud (or silently) the follow invocation:

**'To the Highest of the High please place a large gilt (golden and carved) box around the house and gardens, trapping any human-manifested thought forms or life forms inside ensuring that the golden box is mirrored on the inside.'**

**Step 3:** Visualise or ask for the sides, top and floor to move in, just like an Indiana Jones movie. Gradually, the pressure will build up inside the box until it cannot be retained any longer, the lid will burst open shooting all the detrimental forms straight up into the light where they are disposed of in an appropriate fashion.

**Step 4:** See the golden box shrink until it fits into the hand of Archangel Azriel who then, when asked, will take it to the light and dispose of it appropriately.

**Step 5:** Then to finish, either say out loud or in your head the following:

**'I ask that an ultra-fine mesh net of light and love is pulled through the house (above the house, below the ground and to either side as**

appropriate) picking up all residue left behind by human manifested thought forms and life forms. I then ask that the net is taken to the light and disposed of appropriately, leaving the house in peace, balance, and harmony for the family. I ask that the healing takes place not only in this dimension but all other dimensions that are similarly affected.'

**Step 6:** Dowse to check that the house is now free of detrimental energy forms, just in case there are more layers that need to be cleared.

This method has changed slightly since my first book. I was teaching a course a few years ago and one of the attendees, a very sensitive lad, found two thought forms in his home. He set about removing them in the original manner, but as the walls began to close in, he started to look very uncomfortable. He actually felt the pain and anguish of the thought forms as they were turned inside out, this happened naturally as they saw their reflection in the mirrors, just before they went to the light.

I do not like any being to suffer as I carry out a healing, therefore I wanted to devise another, kinder, method of removing them without causing any hurt or anxiety.

# 4. Lower Animal Life Forms

These will have been removed at the same time as the detrimental or inappropriate attachments, using the Ultra-Fine Mesh Net of Light and Love. But please dowse and check that they are indeed cleared and have gone to the light.

# 5. Sorcery/Black Magic

The healing needed to clear any black magic depends on how bad the problem is. If it is between 0 and -5, then flooding the problem with light and love (heavenly healing) should work – whilst asking for all the dark energies there to be taken to the light. However, if it is -6 and above then do the following.

**Step 1:** Dowse to ensure your psychic protection is in place.

**Step 2:** Connect with your higher self, or spirit guide. They will be your intermediary, to keep the energy at arm's length.

**Step 3:** Visualise a courtroom scene with Archangel Michael as judge and jury. The person or persons who created the problem are in the dock; (the offender) and your higher self is the prosecutor, sitting with his/her client stating their case. It is a matter of you plea-bargaining for the injured, innocent party, asking the accused to admit their guilt.

**Step 4:** Once they have admitted their part in creating the problem, ask Archangel Michael to remove the offending energies, sending them to the light where they are disposed of appropriately.

**Step 5:** Dowse to make sure the sorcery or black magic traces have been cleared. In rare cases, you might have to go to the top court and enlist the Highest of the High to help. Go through the same procedure, asking that the person be found guilty and made to clear up the dark energies that they left behind.

**Step 6:** Once completed, ask that all parties (both the innocent and the guilty) are flooded with light and love, placing them all in bubbles of white light, for the guilty party, place mirrors on the inside and for the innocent, place the mirrors on the outside.

The healing gives absolution to the perpetrator.

**Step 7:** Dowse to check that the house is now free of the effects of black magic/sorcery, just in case there are more layers that need to be cleared.

5

# 6. Spirit Lines

To heal a detrimental spirit line, carry out the following exercise:

**Step 1:** Dowse to check your protection is in place.

**Step 2:** Then, just like carrying out a soul rescue recite the following invocations:

**'To the Highest of the High, please shine a beam of beautiful white light in front of each lost soul and show each of the spirits a vision of what awaits them, in Heaven. Their own idea of perfection.'**

**Step 3:** Recite:

**'Ladies and gentlemen, please do not be afraid by this direct form of communication as I have been granted special dispensation to talk to you today, to help you to continue your interrupted journey into the light.**

**An 'Ultra-Fine Mesh Net of Light and Love' has been pulled through your auric fields removing any attachments and cutting any physical and psychic cords, leading to you or from you, that held you back, so you can now move through when you are ready.**

**You have been shown a vision of what awaits you, it is perfection, a true paradise, certainly far better than staying here on this cold grey mundane earth plane. It is a beautiful place to be, and there**

are many people are waiting for you to arrive with open arms and unconditional love.

Should you wish anyone from your past to be with you now, to hold your hand or just help guide you on your journey, call their name and they will appear beside you.

There will be no retribution for anything that you have done whilst on this earth plane, or that has been done to you, as this has been part of your life's plan. This will be explained to you, once you arrive.

I therefore invite you now to move into the light, and to be with your family, friends, loved ones, comrades, colleagues and pets once again. Amen.'

**Step 4:** Check to see if they have all moved on, and again in a few days, as there may be a few stranglers left to help move through.

**Step 5:** If any of the souls have not gone to the light it may be there is a controlling spirit involved, dowse to see if this is the case. If so, you will need to find a way of encouraging them to move through before the other souls are released. Talking to them individually can often work; egos survive even after death.

Repeat the Soul Rescue Invocation and dowse to see if they have gone this time, if not, dig deeper to find out why. In most cases, it will be a matter of reassuring them that there will no retribution for anything that they have done whilst on the Earth plane.

**Step 6:** I rarely divert lines, preferring to heal and harmonise them, but spirit lines are one of the exceptions to this rule. Once all the spirits have gone, say out loud:

'I ask that the line is flooded with light and love, removing any detrimental energy patterns, disposing of them into the Universe, and leaving the line in peace, balance and harmony for all time. I also ask that the line is now appropriately diverted from all houses and buildings that it has affected detrimentally, leaving it to run harmlessly through gardens, and along roads and footpaths. I ask that the healing takes place not only in this dimension but all other dimensions that are similarly affected.'

**Step 8:** Finish off this exercise by stating the following:

'I ask that any doorways opened expectedly or unexpectedly during my dowsing/healing work are now firmly closed, and that any residue left behind by the lost souls passing through is now removed and taken into the light, leaving the house in peace, balance and harmony.'

6

# Earth Energies

# 7. Water Veins/ Underground Streams

7 Now we are entering the geomancy stage of the healing process. Looking at and working with the energy patterns of the Earth, helping bring a balance to this topsy-turvy world.

I suggest, initially, that you work on the water veins one at a time; however, as you get more practiced, you can begin to tackle them as a whole.

**Step 1:** Dowse to check your protection is in place.

**Step 2:** Visualise the vein being flooded with light and love along its entire length, depth, and breadth.

**Step 3:** Recite the following:

'I ask that all detrimental energies contained in the water vein to be removed and disposed of appropriately into the Universe.'

**Step 4:** Once that has been carried out, flood the water vein with light and love once again, saying:

'I now ask that the water vein be left in peace, balance, and harmony for all living things for all time.'

**Step 5:** Recite the following:

'To the Highest of the High, I now ask that this water vein be moved away from my home, both energetically and physically, and all other houses that it affects detrimentally, as appropriate, for it to now flow harmlessly beneath gardens, pathways and roads, and to leave the stream in peace, balance and harmony for all living things for all time. I ask that the healing takes place not only in this dimension but all other dimensions that are similarly affected.'

I use the words 'as appropriate' because certain occupants may need the water vein or veins to continue flowing beneath their homes, requiring the energy that they create, good or bad. Only Upstairs knows why.

It normally takes between twenty-four and forty-eight hours for the water veins to move from their current position to their new location.

**Step 6:** Repeat Steps 2-5 for each remaining water vein.

**Step 7:** The next day dowse to see how far the water veins have moved.

The healing that you have sent will travel for miles along the diverted water vein, into streams, rivers and finally the sea, travelling around the planet. How cool is that?

# 8. Any other detrimental water source

Whether you have found an area of trapped ancient water, a covered well, a blindhead spring, an underground lake or a secondary spring, you will need to follow this process to heal and harmonise.

**Step 1:** Dowse to check your psychic protection is in place.

**Step 2:** Recite the following:

**'To the Highest of the High I ask that every molecule of water within the trapped water/ancient water is flooded with healing light from Spirit above and the Earth below. I ask that healing is sent to the source of the water, and all detrimental and inappropriate energy patterns contained within it are removed and disposed of into the Universe. I ask that the healing takes place not only in this dimension but all other dimensions that are similarly affected.'**

**Step 3:** For a blindhead spring/water dome I request the following:

**'To the Highest of the High I ask that the energy particles flowing/rising from the halted blindhead spring are flooded with light and love removing all the detrimental and inappropriate energy patterns contained within it, which are then dispose of appropriately into the Universe. I ask that the healing takes place not only in this dimension but all other dimensions that are similarly affected.'**

**Step 4:** For a secondary spring running beneath the home, I use the following invocation:

'To the Highest of the High, please flood both the secondary spring and energy patterns emitting from it with light and love, taking the detrimental energy patterns into the light and disposing of them appropriately. Leaving the spring and water in peace, balance, and harmony for all living things for all time. I ask that the healing takes place not only in this dimension but all other dimensions that are similarly affected.'

8

# 9. Earth Energy Lines

If there is more than one earth line, focus on healing one at a time until you gain in experience, then in time you can heal them all in one go.

**Step 1:** Dowse to check your protection is in place.

**Step 2:** Visualise the earth energy line being flooded with light and love along its entire length, depth, and breadth.

**Step 3:** Recite the following:

**'To the Highest of the High, please remove all detrimental human emotion and earth energy problems from this line and from all the places it runs through on its journey around the world, disposing of them appropriately into the Universe, leaving the earth energy line in peace, balance and harmony for all living things for all time. I ask that the healing takes place not only in this dimension but all other dimensions that are similarly affected.'**

**Step 4:** Once that has been carried out, ask that the earth energy line is once again flooded with light and love, for it to be left in peace, balance and harmony for all living things for all time.

**Step 5:** Repeat steps 2 – 4 for all remaining earth energy lines.

# 10. Energy Channels

**Step 1:** Dowse to check your psychic protection is in place.

**Step 2:** Visualise each energy channels being flooded with light and love along their entire length, breadth and depth, and recite the following:

**'To the Highest of the High, please send a healing white light along the whole length of each energy channel, removing all the detrimental human emotion and earth energy problems contained within them. Spreading the healing light into each home they run through, each sacred and holy site, and any water course they interact with. I also ask that anything that has been dislodged is taken and disposed of into the light. I ask that the healing takes place not only in this dimension but all other dimensions that are similarly affected.'**

**Step 3:** See the channels being flooded once again with light and love, and being left in peace, balance, and harmony for all living things, for all time.

# 11. Fault Lines

I deal with fault lines in a similar way as the energy channels above as they contain comparable energy patterns within them. Both tend to run through or close to holy and/or sacred sites therefore can pick up a lot of detrimental human emotion as well as earth energy problems. But the wording of the invocation is slightly different.

**Step 1:** Dowse to check your protection is in place.

**Step 2:** Visualise the fault line being flooded with light and love along the entire length, breadth and depth, and recite the following:

**'To the Highest of the High I ask that a healing white light is sent along the entire length of the fault line, removing all the detrimental human emotion and earth energy problems contained within it, spreading the healing light into each home it runs through each sacred and holy site and any water course it interacts with. I ask that anything that has been dislodged is taken and disposed of into the light. I also ask that the fault line is left in peace, balance and harmony for all living things for all time. I ask that the healing takes place not only in this dimension but all other dimensions that are similarly affected.'**

**Step 3:** See the fault line being flooded once again with light and love, and ask that it be left in peace, balance, and harmony for all living things, for all time.

# 12. Dynamic Energy Lines

**Step 1:** Dowse to check your protection is in place.

**Step 2:** If you found any spirits attached to the line, carry out the soul rescue/spirit release invocation, then dowse to make sure that they have gone to the light.

**Step 3:** Visualise the dynamic energy line being flooded with light and love along its entire length, depth, and breadth.

**Step 4:** Recite the following:

**'To the Highest of the High I ask that a healing white light is sent along the entire length of the dynamic energy line, that each band of energy is being healed by removing all the detrimental human emotion and earth energy problems contained within it, spreading the healing light into each home it runs through, each sacred and holy site and any water course it interacts with. I ask that anything that has been dislodged is taken and disposed of into the light. I also ask that each of the energetic bands contained within the dynamic energy line is left in peace, balance and harmony for all living things for all time. I ask that the healing takes place not only in this dimension but all other dimensions that are similarly affected.'**

**Step 5:** Dowse to check that the house is now free of detrimental energy from the dynamic energy lines.

# 13. Human Intent Lines

**Step 1:** Dowse to check your protection is in place.

**Step 2:** Recite the following:

**'I ask that a divine white light is sent to each of the holy or sacred sites that the human intent line interacts with, removing all the detrimental human emotion and earth energy problems that might exist, taking them into the Universe where they are disposed of appropriately. Once each site has been cleared, I ask that divine light is once again sent to each area leaving them all in peace, balance and harmony for all time. I ask that the healing takes place not only in this dimension but all other dimensions that are similarly affected.'**

**Step 3:** If you found that someone has been 'dirtying the line' on purpose, send healing to them (clear attachments etc.) then place them in a bubble of white light that is mirrored on the inside so that both their detrimental thoughts and actions are reflected inward, but please ensure that this is done with unconditional love.

**Step 4:** Dowse to check that the house is now free of detrimental energy from the human intent lines.

13

# 14. Energy Spirals

**Step 1:** Dowse to ensure your protection is in place.

**Step 2:** If there is more than one spiral, until you are confident enough to clear them all in once go, recite the following for each one in turn:

'**I ask the Highest of the High that a healing white light from above slowly moves downwards following the direction of the spin (clockwise or counter-clockwise), disappearing into the earth, where the detrimental energies are dispersed. Then a healing white light now rises from the earth, moving slowly upwards cleansing the spiral once again, finally connecting with the Universe, and dispersing any further detrimental energy. I ask that the spiral is now fully cleansed and harmonised leaving it in peace, balance, and harmony for all living things for all time. I ask that the healing takes place not only in this dimension but all other dimensions that are similarly affected.**'

**Step 3:** Dowse to check that the spirals are still there and are now beneficial to you and the family. They will be perfect to meditate within and to energise yourself.

14

**Step 4:** Repeat step 2 and 3 for any remaining spirals.

# 15. Energetic Sink Holes

**Step 1:** Dowse to ensure your protection is in place.

**Step 2:** Recite the following:

'**To the Highest of the High I ask that any detrimental, inappropriate energies or beings that may have come though the sink hole are now returned to their own dimensions and healing sent to them as they move through. Any further detrimental energy that may be left behind should also be returned. Once that is done, I ask that a cap or plug of light and love be placed in or over the sink hole sealing it for all time. I ask that the healing takes place not only in this dimension but all other dimensions that are similarly affected.**'

**Step 3:** Dowse to check the energetic sink hole is sealed, and that the area is now clear of detrimental energies.

# 16. Reversal Points

**Step 1:** Dowse to ensure your protection is in place.

**Step 2:** Recite the following:

**'To the Highest of the High I first ask that any detrimental energies caused by covering the reversal point be taken away and disposed of appropriately into the Universe and that the area affected is flooded with light and love. I further ask that a spiritual manhole cover is placed over the reversal point, then a light skim of light and love (spiritual plaster) to seal it completely for all time. I ask that the healing takes place not only in this dimension but all other dimensions that are similarly affected.'**

**Step 3:** Dowse to check the reversal points are now sealed and are no longer detrimental.

16

# 17. Emotional Energy Areas (Human Conflict)

**Step 1:** Dowse to ensure your protection is in place.

**Step 2:** We will now clear items 17 and 24 using the ultra-fine mesh net of light and love. Recite the following:

**'To the Highest of the High I ask that as this ultra-fine mesh net of light and love is being pulled through the house (above the house, below the ground and to either side as appropriate) it clears all emotional energy areas, all bed patterns, and all power artefacts of their detrimental energies. I ask that the net is then taken to the light and disposed of appropriately, leaving the house in peace, balance, and harmony for myself and the family. I ask that the healing takes place not only in this dimension but all other dimensions that are similarly affected.'**

**Step 3:** Dowse to check that each area has been cleared by the net, if you find anything lingering, ask for the net to be pulled through the house again, taking away any remaining residue.

**Step 4:** If there is a very detrimental area in the house it may need extra or individual work. It could have been caused by a murder that took place many years ago, a rape or possibly a suicide. Check how detrimental it is. If -7 and upwards check to see if there is a spirit attached to that location or item of furniture, if so, help them go to the light. Then use the net once again.

17

# 18. Psychic Cords

When dealing with psychic cords you need to be on your guard. Once they have been cut or severed it is very important that you check again in a few days' time, to make sure they have not reattached. The person responsible for attaching the cords in the first place may well be aware that something is missing or changed, probably a subconscious reaction. It may result in you suddenly receiving a communication from them, whether by text, email or telephone call. If that happens, check again to make sure that you are clear.

You can choose from the following two methods to clear psychic cords:

## Method 1: Archangel Michael and his Sword of Light and Truth

**Step 1:** Ensure your psychic protection is in place.

**Step 2:** Visualise the two people connected by a silver thread or threads standing in front of Archangel Michael, one to the left of him and the other to the right. See the cords that join them together and ask Michael to cut them with his sword. Ask that the first cut is where the cord is attached to yourself or the person that you are healing, the second cut is where the cord is attached to the other person, the third and final cut is to sever them completely.

Ask that Michael to take all the fractured pieces to the light and dispose

18

339

of them appropriately.

**Step 3:** Then surround each person in a bubble of white light placing mirrors both on the inside of the bubble as well as the outside. Don't forget that it might have been you who attached the cord so both parties need to be protected from any cords that might re-attach in the short term.

**Step 4:** Dowse to check that all cords have now been cut and cleared, both to the front and back chakras.

**Step 5:** Just to reiterate, please check again in a few days, making sure that you or they are still clear, especially if the person has been in communication. The chances are that they have reconnected the cord or cords. If they have reattached run through the procedure again.

If it keeps happening, then I would carry out a healing on the person involved, using either the spiritual wall or the ultra-fine mesh net of light and love, removing all and any attachments or spirits that may be affecting their behaviour.

## Method 2: Floating Bubble

**Step 1:** Visualise yourself (or member of the family) standing on a cliff top overlooking the sea with far-reaching views. It is a beautiful and warm sunny day with the occasional cloud passing by. The person who has attached the cords to you is enclosed in a multi-coloured bubble floating in front of you.

**Step 2:** See the cords leading from them to you. Take a pair of scissors (or use your fingers in a cutting motion) and cut the cord or cords joining the two of you together and then forcibly blow the bubble away from you, watching it slowly disappear from sight.

**Step 3:** Put yourself and the person you have cleared, in a bubble of white light as above, should the person reattach the cord, carry out the visualisation again.

18

# 19. Dimensional Portals

**Step 1:** Ensure your psychic protection is in place.

**Step 2:** Visualise the Archangels with large nets (rather like the Ultra-Fine Mesh Net of Light and Love) capturing all the undesirable and detrimental beings and energies that may have come through the open portal, returning them to their own dimensions.

**Step 3:** Dowse to make sure they have all gone, then ask that the spiritual door is firmly shut, turn a sacred key in the lock and finally put a skim of light and love (spiritual plaster) over it, asking that it be sealed for all time.

**Step 4:** Then pull an ultra-fine mesh net of light and love through the house once again to clear away any residue that may have been left behind in their passing by stating:

**'To the Highest of the High I ask that as the ultra-fine mesh net of light and love is being pulled through the house (above the house, below the ground and to either side as appropriate) it clears all the residue left behind by any beings from other dimensions. I ask that the net is then taken to the light and disposed of appropriately, leaving the house in peace, balance, and harmony for myself and the family. I ask that the healing takes place not only in this dimension but all other dimensions that are similarly affected.'**

**Step 3:** Dowse to check the dimensional portal is now sealed and is no longer detrimental.

# 20. Illness Trigger Points

**Step 1:** Ensure your psychic protection is in place.

**Step 2:** Having the origin of the problem in front of you as you work through this healing section will help. Once the date, time, place, and cause has been found, then it is time to work on the cure.

**Step 3:** You need to visualise the scene, perhaps running it through your head like a sepia movie. As you do, we need to carry out a clearing on all parties. Place each of the individuals involved in their own private divine white light waiting room ready to move through the spiritual wall.

**Step 4:** When they are ready, move them through the wall reciting the following:

'To the Highest of the High, as each person walks through the spiritual wall I ask that their auric fields and physical body are cleared of all detrimental and inappropriate attachments that were with them at that time, all lower animal life forms, including their seeds and tentacles, any illness trigger points, all human manifested thought forms and life forms, all detrimental psychic and physical cords to be cut, clearing all worries and concerns, any miasms and detrimental family DNA, any cancers and tumours, any past, present, parallel and simultaneous life traumas or upsets, all detrimental parental patterning, all parasites and any other detrimental energies that were inappropriate to them at that stage in their lives and that the healing

**takes place not only in this dimension but all other dimensions that are similarly affected.'**

**Step 4:** Then I would dowse to make sure that this was successful. I would also ask if there was any further healing that might need to be carried out. This may be in the form of forgiveness, or understanding, by the person who was affected.

20

# 21. Consecrated Ground

**Step 1:** Dowse to ensure your psychic protection is in place.

**Step 2:** If we are dealing with an old church, chapel or a sacred place we first need to ask permission, from Upstairs, to clear away the energy imprints left behind by years of worship, effectively deconsecrating the building or land.

Recite the following:

**'To the Highest of the High I request permission to deconsecrate this land/building for the highest good of those living upon it.'**

Wait a few moments, then dowse to see if you have permission. If you do, go to step 4. If not, go to step 3.

**Step 3:** If permission is not given, ask if there are any lost souls to rescue first and if there are, follow the soul rescue/spirit release method. Once they have gone to the light, clear away any residue and also any detrimental earth energy patterns and stuck human emotion using the ultra-fine mesh net of light and love. Once this has been carried out, ask again if you can deconsecrate the building and land.

If you get permission this time, then go to step 4. If permission is still not given, you will need to dowse again, asking further questions to determine why. It may be the wrong time of the week/month or year, the moon phase may not be correct or there may have to be forgiveness sought for a past act. Once you have found out why then move on.

**Step 4:** Recite the following:

'**To the Highest of the High I ask that all energetic patterns from the past, including any and all religious memories, all detrimental human emotion and any earth energies associated with these religious practices, are taken into the Universe and disposed of appropriately. Deconsecrating the buildings and land, returning the energies to normal living levels for now and at all times in the future. I also ask that the healing takes place not only in this dimension but all other dimensions that are similarly affected.**'

**Step 5:** Dowse to check that the land/building is now deconsecrated and cleared of any energetic imprints of previous use.

# 22. Curses and Spells

**Step 1:** Check your psychic protection is in place.

**Step 2:** Ask your higher self and Spirit to check that the spells can be cleared and/or lifted. You will more than likely get an affirmative answer.

**Step 3:** Ask for your Higher Self to work directly with Archangel Michael and the Higher Self of the person responsible for casting the spell or curse. You are acting as an intermediary, plea bargaining for the person who is the recipient of these detrimental thoughts and energies. Having run through all the questions, you should already know the reason why the spell was cast in the first place and by whom.

**Step 4:** Either in your head, or speaking out loud, you put your case forward, saying why you feel the person on the receiving end has been wronged and why the spell or curse should now be lifted. It will be a one-sided conversation.

**Step 5:** Once you have put your case forward, dowse to make sure that the curse or spell and been lifted. If it has not, ask why. Perhaps there is a lost soul that needs to be helped before the curse can be lifted, or you may need to send healing (or understanding) to the person who caused the problem. You may have to release some trapped elementals or remove/clear the detrimental emotion in the house. Or all the above. Find out what else needs to happen, then ask again for the spell or curse to be lifted.

**Step 6:** Dowse to check it has been lifted now.

**Step 7:** Send unconditional love to the person that set the spell or curse, we do not want to fight fire with fire, this can diffuse the chances of it happening again.

**Step 8:** Check again in a week or so to make sure it has been cleared.

22

# 23. Psychic Attack

**Step 1:** Check your psychic protection.

**Step 2:** Using the Spiritual Wall method, visualise yourself (or the member of your family member who is affected) in their own private spiritual waiting room, and the perpetrator in theirs. Then when ready see the affected person moving through the holy wall, reciting the following invocation:

**'To the Highest of the High please remove all detrimental energy patterns leading to, and resulting from the psychic attack, whether it comes from conscious or subconscious thought. I also ask that this healing light moves through their body, chakras and aura, cleansing them 100%. Leaving them in peace, balance and harmony. I ask that the healing takes place not only in this dimension but all other dimensions that are similarly affected.'**

For the person that is sending the detrimental thoughts recite the following:

**'To the Highest of the High I ask that as this man/woman walks through the spiritual wall, all detrimental thoughts and attachments are removed, and they are taken to the light and disposed of in an appropriate fashion. I ask that any jealousy, envy, greed, upset, or malicious thoughts that led to them psychically attacking (name), be cleared and for their mind, body and spirit to be left in peace,**

balance and harmony. I ask that the healing takes place not only in this dimension but all other dimensions that are similarly affected.'

**Step 3:** State out loud:

'To the Highest of the High, please place (name) in a bubble of white light for as long as is necessary to keep them fully protected. The bubble is mirrored on the outside, reflecting any further detrimental thoughts being sent their way, being returned to the sender with unconditional love.'

**Step 4:** Recite the following:

'To the Highest of the High, please place the perpetrator in a bubble of white light, mirrored on the inside to stop any further detrimental thoughts from escaping. These are reflected and returned to him/her with unconditional love.'

**Step 5:** Forgiveness and understanding is also part of the healing process. To forgive the person who attacked you and to understand why it happened.

**Step 6:** Dowse to check that everyone is free of the detrimental energies of psychic attack.

# 24. Power Artefacts

These will have been healed at the same time as the emotional energy areas (17), but it is a good idea to dowse to ensure that they are indeed clear.

If one, or more, of the artefacts is not cleared, check to make sure that the object does not have a spirit attached to it, if it does, carry out a soul rescue. Once done use the ultra-fine mesh net of light and love once again making sure that all the detrimental energy patterns are taken to the light. As a fail-safe you can ask that each artefact is flooded with light and love, being left in peace, balance and harmony.

# 25. Place Memory

**Step 1:** Check your psychic protection is in place.

**Step 2:** Dowse to see if the place memory area (or areas) has any lost souls or possibly life forms or thought forms attached to them. If they do, work through the soul rescue/spirit release method and then clear away the thought or life forms.

**Step 3:** State out loud:

**'To the Highest of the High I ask that as the ultra-fine mesh net of light and love is being pulled through the house (above, below the ground and to either side as appropriate) it picks up all the residue from any lost souls or life and thought forms attached to the place memory, and that it clears all detrimental energy patterns that caused the place memory to come into existence. I ask that the net is taken to the light and disposed of appropriately, leaving the house in peace, balance, and harmony for the family. I ask that the healing takes place not only in this dimension but all other dimensions that are similarly affected.'**

**Step 4:** If extra layers were indicated in your questioning, you should now dowse to see if you can heal them straight away. Otherwise, you may need to wait a few days or weeks to do so, this can take time, as it depends on how deep or detrimental the area was and what caused it to come into existence.

**Step 5:** Flood the affected area with light and love, leaving it in peace, balance, and harmony for ever more.

# 26. Interdimensional Place Memory

**Step 1:** Check your psychic protection is in place.

**Step 2:** Dowse to see if the interdimensional place memory has any lost souls to deal with first, there may even be a life or thought forms to clear. If so, complete the lost soul/spirit release method and then move on to removing the thought or life forms.

**Step 3:** Recite the following:

'**To the Highest of the High I ask that as the ultra-fine mesh net of light and love is being pulled through the house (above, below the ground and to either side as appropriate) it picks up all the residue from any lost souls or life/thought forms attached to the interdimensional place memory, and that it clears all detrimental energy patterns caused by the interdimensional place memory. I ask that all detrimental energies be taken back to their own dimension where they are disposed of appropriately, leaving the house in peace, balance, and harmony for the family. I ask that the healing takes place not only in this dimension but all other dimensions that are similarly affected.**'

**Step 4:** If further layers were indicated in your questioning, dowse to see if you are able to heal them now, or if you need to check again in a few days.

**Step 5:** Flood the affected area with light and love, leaving it in peace, balance, and harmony for ever more.

**Step 6:** And finally recite the following:

**'To the Highest of the High, please reinforce the veil/barrier between the dimensions, to strengthen and reinforce the area or patch that allowed the detrimental energy patterns to 'bleed' or pass through. Leaving it sealed for all time.'**

26

# 27. Vows or Contracts

By working through all the questions, finding out dates, your sex at the time and what the vow entailed will make it so much easier to rescind the vow or contract in this lifetime. Knowing this information helps you to start the healing process.

**Step 1:** Check your psychic protection is in place.

**Step 2:** Visualise yourself as the person who made the vow, hear yourself speaking the words.

**Step 3:** Recite the following invocation:

**'To the Highest of the High I ask that all and any vows or contracts that I have generated in any lifetime, whether in this dimension or another are now revoked and fully annulled. I also request that healing is sent to any other person or persons that may have been affected by my actions.'**

**Step 4:** If you are not the person who made the vow or contract then you need to ask them to say the above words. It is good enough for them to read the words, but even better if they are prepared to say them out loud. You may suddenly feel a rush of emotion, whether sadness or elation as the vow or contract is fully lifted. This is part of the healing process, just allow the emotions to come to the surface and give thanks.

**Step 5:** Dowse to check all vows and contracts have been cleared.

# 28. Fractured/Torn Souls

**Step 1:** Make sure your psychic protection is in place.

**Step 2:** Using the Spiritual Wall method, visualise the person with the torn soul sitting in the waiting room, then walking through the spiritual wall into the divine white light room, this removes all the attachments that may have entered the body or aura via the tear.

**Step 3:** Summon one of the Archangels (the choice is yours as to which one) to help. I normally invoke Michael. Recite the following:

**'Archangel Michael, please mend the tear (in the aura) or restore any part of the soul that might have been fractured. Once fully repaired please put a bubble of white light around the newly repaired soul, keeping it protected until it has had a chance to fully heal itself.** (This normally takes two to three days.)

**Step 4:** Send healing back to the time the soul became fractured or torn, and also to the person/event that caused it to happen. Then ask Archangel Michael for the person to be left in peace, balance, and harmony.

**Step 5:** Dowse again, in a few days, to check if the tear or fracture has been mended. Further healing work may be needed, possibly more attachments need clearing before you can fully repair the soul.

Some people will feel different when this healing has been carried out, but many do not. There are no rules when it comes to soul repair or retrieval. But it will be beneficial, there is no doubt.

# 29. Stress/Disturbance Lines (Man-made)

**Step 1:** Check your psychic protection is in place.

**Step 2:** Working on one line at a time (until you become more experienced) visualise the stress line being flooded with light and love along its entire length, depth, and breadth.

**Step 3:** Recite the following:

'**To the Highest of the High I ask that all detrimental energies contained in this line be removed and disposed of appropriately into the Universe.**'

**Step 4:** Once that has been carried out, flood the stress line once again with light and love, asking the following:

'**I ask that the stress line now be left in peace, balance, and harmony for all living things for all time. I ask that the healing takes place not only in this dimension but all other dimensions that are similarly affected.**'

**Step 5:** I also send a healing light to the area where the stress lines were created. If because of physical abuse between spouses, then send healing to them both. Use the Spiritual Wall method, asking that all detrimental and inappropriate energies be removed, including any attachments, and then sent to the Universe leaving the couple in peace, balance and harmony.

356

If it was created by GM crops, spraying the land with chemicals, mining, or digging foundations for new builds, or by hospitals or other buildings that contain detrimental energies, you can use the ultra-fine mesh net of light and love, pulling the net through the affected area, asking that all detrimental and inappropriate energies be removed, and then taken to the Universe leaving the location in peace, balance and harmony.

**Step 6:** Dowse to make sure that the line has been cleared. If it has not after your first attempt, try sending healing once again, to the people concerned and the area the problem originated from. The deeper and more detrimental the energies are the more difficult they can be too clear in one go, layers may well exist, and as they rise to the surface, continue to clear them away until all the problems have gone.

29

# 30. Karmic Problems – Simultaneous Life Trauma

To heal a trauma in a simultaneous life, we are going to visit the place in time where you (or a family member) experienced the trauma that is affecting this life.

If easier you can visualise it as a direct timeline (you, living a past life) or as a dimensional life (all lives at the same time). It doesn't make a difference how you visualise it; healing is healing.

Even if you are not fully sure, or do not want to know what the trauma was, purely by setting your intent should prove to be enough. Sometimes it is better not to remember and just ask for the appropriate healing to take place. The choice is yours.

**Step 1:** Ensure your psychic protection is in place.

**Step 2:** Sit quietly, and for at least ten minutes, clear your mind of day-to-day dross and think about the task ahead. Soft spiritual music can sometimes help you achieve a peaceful and calm mind; you owe it to yourself to take your time as the whole experience can be quite moving. I would suggest that a box of tissues is close by, just in case.

**Step 3:** Call upon your higher self to be your intermediary for the procedure, along with the other party's higher self. Call upon Archangel Michael to help the process move forward smoothly; he will oversee fair play.

358

**Step 4:** With your notes from the diagnosis, re-run the story of the trauma through your head rather like a Hollywood movie – do not worry about the colours, you can work in sepia.

Using the example of my life as the alchemist, when I died an early death due to unhappiness; I would start by sending healing to all the members of my family, asking for their forgiveness, and to explain why I was so unhappy and died so young. That basically, I died from a broken heart. Then I would send healing to myself in that lifetime. Time is not linear so it can be done. I would clear away any attachments that might have been connected to my unhappiness.

**Step 5:** Carry out the same process for your next reincarnation or dimensional life until you finally reach your current life where you will need to ascertain whether or not you have already made a similar or related mistake, perhaps to a lesser degree, that needs healing.

**Step 6:** Once all the lives affected have been healed, check to make sure that all is well.

**Step 7:** You might need to go back and carry out a further healing, particularly if it was a difficult past/dimensional life issue; you could call upon one of your ancestors to help you. Dowse which one and work with them.

**Step 8:** Finally, ask Archangel Michael to take away all the detrimental energy that you have generated throughout this life, and/or past incarnations, disposing of them all appropriately into the Universe.

30

# 30a. Karmic Problems – Parallel Life Trauma

**Step 1:** Ensure your psychic protection is in place.

**Step 2:** Sit quietly, for at least ten minutes, and clear your mind.

**Step 3:** Call upon Archangel Michael to assist you.

**Step 4:** Focus on the parallel life that is causing you the challenges in this current life, picture yourself in that life, with the problem or problems. Ask Archangel Michael to cut any cords leading from you to the difficulties that you are facing, and any cords linking you to that parallel self. Then put your parallel self in a healing bubble of light, so they too can get a reprieve from the detrimental energy. You can ask that they are cleared of any detrimental attachments they may have picked up and also for any emotional issues to be healed.

**Step 5:** When it feels clear, focus on the next parallel life, but only if you have detected that there is another one causing you issues. Carry out the same exercise.

**Step 6:** Once all of the lives affected have been cleared and healed, dowse to make sure that all is well. Ask Archangel Michael to then strengthen the boundaries between the different dimensions, so that each one does not detrimentally affect another. This stops any domino effect occurring.

# 31. Detrimental Implants

The healing needed really depends on what type of implants you have found:

## Reiki:

If they are the incorrect or corrupted Reiki symbols, then I would suggest going back to the Master who attuned you, asking that they be removed. Then to be reattuned using fresh and uncorrupted symbols. Or ask the 'Powers that be' if there is something that you can do to help yourself, with their assistance. If they say yes, then follow these steps:

**Step 1:** Check that your psychic protection is in place.

**Step 2:** Ask that the corrupted or incorrect symbols are removed from your aura and, in some cases, your body may have also been affected. The spiritual wall is very useful for this exercise. As you move from the 'waiting room' through the wall to the divine white light room the other side recite the following:

**'To the Highest of the High I ask that as I (or name) walk through the spiritual wall that any and all corrupted or incorrect Reiki symbols are removed from my aura and physical body and are then taken to the light, leaving me clear of any past problems associated with them. I ask that the healing takes place not only in this dimension but all other dimensions that are similarly affected.'**

**Step 3:** I would then ask if it is appropriate for the Highest of the High or one of the Archangels to re-attune you. If so then ask them to place the correct healing symbols back into your aura, enabling you to channel the pure Reiki energy once again, not just for yourself but others too.

## Surgical Implants:

If something has been implanted via a surgical method, such as a pacemaker, stent, a metal pin or new joint, then follow these steps:

**Step 1:** Ensure your psychic protection is in place.

**Step 2:** Flood the implant/s with light and love asking that all detrimental energy patterns be removed and sent to the light.

**Step 3:** Dowse to check after the healing has taken place to make sure that you have covered and cleared everything that needed to be dealt with. You can, if you wish, flood the article once again with light and love asking that it be left in peace, balance and harmony with you and your body.

## Off-World (ET):

If you find any off-world implants, then follow this process:

**Step 1:** Ensure your psychic protection is in place.

**Step 2:** Flood the implant/s with light and love (which should help to deactivate them) asking that all the detrimental energy patterns be taken to the light and disposed of appropriately.

**Step 3:** Use the Ultra-Fine Mesh Net of Light and Love, and reciting the following invocation:

**'To the Highest of the High I ask that, as I pull the ultra-fine mesh net of light and love through (name) auric field and physical body that all implants are short-circuited and deactivated, then pass or exit from their body as soon as possible, leaving them in peace, balance and harmony. I also ask that any detrimental energy patterns that have been removed or dislodged are taken to the light and disposed of appropriately. I ask that the healing takes place not only in this dimension but all other dimensions that are similarly affected.'**

362

**Step 4:** Dowse to check you or the person you are working on are now clear of any detrimental energies caused by off-world implants.

# 32. Toxic Lines

**Step 1:** Check your protection is in place.

**Step 2:** Visualise the toxic line being flooded with light and love along its entire length, depth, and breadth.

**Step 3:** Recite the following:

'**To the Highest of the High I ask that all detrimental energies contained within this toxic line be removed and disposed of appropriately into the Universe.**'

**Step 4:** Once that has been carried out, flood the toxic line again with light and love, and recite the following statement:

'**I now ask that the toxic line be left in peace, balance, and harmony for all living things for all time.**'

**Step 5:** Finally, state the following:

'**To the Highest of the High, I ask for healing and forgiveness to be sent to the source of this toxic line. May the place and each person involved be cleared of all detrimental and inappropriate energies and then to be left in peace, balance and harmony. I also ask that all residue from the toxic line be cleared from this home and any other homes that it affects detrimentally, as appropriate. I ask that the healing takes place not only in this dimension but all other**

**dimensions that are similarly affected.'**

**Step 6:** Then dowse to check if the toxic line has gone, if it has not, flood it with light a final time.

32

# 33. Chakra Alignments and/or Blockages

There are two methods to getting your chakras unblocked and spinning freely again.

## Method One:

**Step 1:** Make sure that your psychic protection is in place.

**Step 2:** Check to see which way each blocked chakra is spinning, you can visualise it, or them, all furred up or rusty, that might make it easier for you to picture. Mentally, or out loud, ask for it to stop spinning. Once it has turn it psychically in the opposite direction (normally three full turns are needed to dislodge the blockage), then start it spinning once again in the correct direction of rotation.

**Step 3:** Recite the following invocation

**'To the Highest of the High I ask that the blocked chakra (or chakras) are now flooded with light and love, and that all the 'junk' that has been dislodged is taken to the light, disposed of appropriately, to leave all the chakra fully cleared, spinning for maximum health and in balance with my mind, body and soul.'**

**Step 4:** Dowse to check that they are now spinning freely and are working optimally.

## Method Two:

**Step 1:** Dowse to ensure your psychic protection is in place.

**Step 2:** Take three deep breaths and relax, listen to the rhythm of your breathing. In – out, in – out, gradually start to introduce a bright golden colour into your in-breath. See this golden light filling up your lungs and as you breathe out begin to let go of your problems. See all your worries, stresses and concerns disappear from your body as black blobs within the golden light.

**Step 3:** After a few minutes, introduce the golden light into your main blocked chakra, imagining it being drawn in on each inhalation and then on the out breath letting go of all the 'emotional junk' and any blockages in the chakra. Keep this going for a few minutes and then gradually begin to work on any other of the chakras that may be blocked.

**Step 4:** You can repeat this as often as you like as it will help keep the chakras in good working order.

## Balancing Chakras:

There are various ways to balance chakras. You can use the breathing method above or you can use the following:

## Pendulum Method:

Working on someone laying in front of you:

**Step 1:** Make sure that your psychic protection is in place.

**Step 2:** Hold the pendulum over the out-of-balance chakra allowing it to spin in whichever direction it wants to, setting your intention as it does so, to clear and stabilise the chakra. You may find that once the healing has been successful the pendulum will stop or reverse direction.

**Step 3:** Repeat this process over each chakra to balance them.

33

## Working on yourself:

**Step 1:** Ensure that your psychic protection is in place.

**Step 2:** Sit comfortably with both feet on the floor and take a few deep breaths — relax and be in touch with your body.

**Step 3:** See a healing beam of light entering your body through the top of your head, moving through to your heart and splitting, moving down each arm, channelling through your hands and finally into your pendulum.

**Step 4:** Hold your pendulum comfortably in front of you and set your intention to work on your feet chakras, you do not have to bend down and hold the pendulum over them. Set the pendulum swinging and let it settle in a circular motion (it does not matter which way) leave it until it either stops or starts swinging the opposite way. Then set your intention to work on your knee chakras then do the same as you work upwards through your base chakra, then sacral, solar plexus, heart, thymus, throat, third eye and finally your crown.

**Step 5:** Once you have worked through the chakras, dowse to make sure that they are now all in balance and that they be left spinning to ensure maximum benefit, health, and protection for you.

# 34. Anything else affecting the house and family (in garden/grounds or close by)

It depends on what you have found as to how you go about healing the problem.

If it's a spirit issue, then use the soul rescue/spirit release invocation in section 1 to help move them into the light, then use the Ultra-Fine Mesh Net of Light and Love method to remove any residue that may be left behind.

If it is earth energy related then use the method described in healing section 9, if perhaps a human intent line then clear the old energy patterns, both the human emotional aspect as well as any earth energy problems (healing section 15). It may be a water vein, if so refer to the healing method that I have described in section 7 and 8.

If it is a neighbour problem, ask for the person or persons to be cleared using the Spiritual Wall method. That should clear them of any attachments that may be causing them to act the way that they are. But do check their house for lost souls and detrimental lines as well.

34

# 35. Fabric of the Building

**Step 1:** Ensure that your psychic protection is in place.

**Step 2:** Use the ultra-fine mesh net of light and love pulling it through the house. Reciting the following invocation:

**'To the Highest of the High I ask that as the ultra-fine mesh net of light and love is being pulled through the house (above, below the ground and to either side as appropriate) it picks up all the detrimental energy that has become trapped within the fabric of the building, and in all the artefacts within the building. I also ask that the net is taken to the light and disposed of appropriately, leaving the house in peace, balance, and harmony for the family. I ask that the healing takes place not only in this dimension but all other dimensions that are similarly affected.'**

**Step 3:** Dowse to make sure that has solved the problem.

**Step 4:** If that has not fully worked, then say the following:

**'Highest of the High, please focus a beam of white light on each of the problematic areas, clearing all the detrimental energies associated with them leaving the house and family in peace, balance and harmony for all time.'**

35

**Step 5:** Dowse again to check if this has worked, or if there are further layers to clear. Depending on how detrimental the energy patterns were will determine whether you may need to carry out a further healing/ clearing. Anything above -6 in detrimental effect will need to be looked at again in a week or so's time, you can dowse to find out the exact day the next healing needs to be carried out.

# 36. Anaesthetic Traces, Inoculations, Vaccinations, Heavy Metals

If your dowsing suggests that you can carry out the healing on yourself, follow the method below.

**Step 1:** Make sure that your psychic protection is in place.

**Step 2:** Recite the following invocation:

**'To the Highest of the High I ask that as an ultra-fine mesh net of light and love is pulled through my body and aura, all of the detrimental effects of anaesthetic traces, vaccinations, inoculations and heavy metals are cleared, whether they be physical or energetic, and anything that has been dislodged or is inappropriate be taken into the light and disposed of in an appropriate fashion. I ask that the healing takes place not only in this dimension but all other dimensions that are similarly affected.'**

**Step 3:** Dowse to check if this has been effective. It may be that you will need carry out the same healing again in a few weeks' time to make sure that all the problems are clear.

If this hasn't been as effective as you wish, then I would recommend you going to see a good homeopath/naturopath who should be able to help you further.

The same applies to heavy metals: there are patches which are placed on your feet that are claimed to remove many of the toxins from your body,

36

and the idea is that they draw out the poisons. I have never used them as I find that the healing process works well for me; however, do look on the internet and carry out some research if you feel that is your best way forward.

Chlorella and Spirulina are two supplements that are used by many people to help rid the body of detrimental toxins and fight off the effects of living in the twenty-first century. They are effective in clearing trace metals found in vegetables, for example. I use them both regularly. There are several books written about these new 'wonder supplements' that are available on the internet, like *The Chlorella Factor* by Mike Adams.

But please be careful as the effects of a cleansing can be very powerful and I would always suggest consulting with a recognised and fully trained naturopath or homeopath before taking any supplements or drastically changing your diet.

36

# 37. Parasites

The late Dr Hulda Clark invented what she referred to as a zapper, a machine that gives out a mild low energy output which kills off detrimental parasites in your body; but it does need to be used on a regular basis. Many people have found it very beneficial; I cannot attest to its effectiveness as I have not tried it myself, but I have had clients who have tried it and have been happy with the results. For further details visit www.huldaclark.com.

My method for dealing with parasites is as follows:

**Step 1:** Ensure your psychic protection is in place.

**Step 2:** Use the Ultra-Fine Mesh Net of Light and Love method by stating the following:

**'To the Highest of the High I ask that as the ultra-fine mesh net of light and love is pulled through my (or name's) body, and that any parasites are cleared away, physically and energetically, to then make sure that anything dislodged or is inappropriate be taken into the light and disposed of in a correct fashion. I ask that the healing takes place not only in this dimension but all other dimensions that are similarly affected.'**

**Step 3:** Dowse to check that the parasites have been dealt with. You may need to use this method several times over the course of a week to clear them all. If you get symptoms of parasite die-off, drink plenty of water to flush toxins out of your system, get plenty of exercise, and ask the Highest of the High to lessen the symptoms where possible.

Removing parasites can be a long process and produce a number of adverse side effects including depression, bloating, and emotional upset, if you prefer a more recognised method of treatment do consult a good naturopath or homeopath who will help you with your diet and supplements to eradicate these light blighters.

# 38. Off-World Interference, Psychic Attack, Psychic Cords

**Step 1:** Ensure your psychic protection is in place.

**Step 2:** Visualise the person and the Off-Worlder connected by the cords standing in front of Archangel Michael, one to the left and the other to the right. See the cords that link them, asking Michael to cut them with his sword or light and truth. The first cut is where the cord attaches to the person you are clearing, the second cut is where the cord originates, the third and final cut is in the middle of the cords, severing them completely.

Then ask Michael to take all the fractured pieces into the light and dispose of them appropriately.

**Step 3:** Surround each person in a bubble of white light, the person that you have cleared with mirrors on the outside to reflect any cords from reattaching. The Off-Worlder with mirrors on the inside to stop them from sending and attaching any further cords.

**Step 4:** Dowse to check that all cords between them have now been severed, to the front of the body, back, above the head and below the feet.

**Step 5:** Depending on how detrimental the cord or cords were, you can dowse to see if they need to be placed in a mirrored pyramid for a few days, if so, visualise that person (family member or yourself) laying on a comfortable bed or sitting in a chair at the centre of the pyramid.

Although the person won't be seen from outside, they will be able to see people walking past, like a two-way mirror. So, that they won't feel isolated and are 100% protected.

**Step 6:** In a few days, dowse to check that they are still cleared. If any cords have reattached go through the process again, but I have never needed to.

# 39. Off-World Lines

The off-world beings who set up these lines originally were unaware that the vibrational energy was going to be detrimental to humans and animals and therefore they are quite happy, if you find such a line, for you to work on it, effectively changing the frequency and only the frequency.

But it's very important that you do not interfere with, change, or stop what they are doing (the energy extraction), as this can and will cause problems for us and them.

**Step 1:** Ensure your psychic protection is in place.

**Step 2:** State the following:

**'To the Highest of the High I ask that the off-world line is now flooded with light and love changing the vibration frequency levels so that it is no longer harmful to life on the Earth, removing all the detrimental patterns, but allowing the line to exist in a beneficial way for both ourselves and its creators. I ask that the healing takes place not only in this dimension but all other dimensions that are similarly affected.'**

**Step 3:** Dowse to check that the line is no longer giving off a detrimental energy.

If you receive the answer that my help is needed to help harmonise the line, do get in touch by emailing me at adrian@dowsingspirits.co.uk.

# 40. Detrimental Planetary Rays

The effects of these rays are very similar to those felt during the cycles of the moon, sometimes they are benevolent, and other times are unsettling, leading to insomnia, vivid dreams, headaches, and mood swings.

Not only do these rays come from our neighbouring planets, but from outside our solar system too. A lot of people feel connected to the Pleiades star system, others to Arcturus and some to Sirius (the Dog Star). Interestingly, they were also worshipped by our ancestors.

When working on nullifying, or clearing, the detrimental energies coming from the stars I always try to find out why we are being affected, then start the healing work. Not all planetary rays are detrimental to us, but they can be very powerful, and if you are not used to dealing with this type of energy, they can become disruptive.

Combining healing energies from the Universe, Mother Earth, Father Sun, and the moon should help with the healing. Just visualise a strong beam of healing white light leading from you to the planet or star system causing the problems, then ask that any and all detrimental energy patterns are removed and disposed of appropriately. To finish, see the planet surrounded by the healing light. Send all the beings there, in physical or ethereal form, unconditional love.

Keep up your psychic protection, the more you do the stronger it becomes. It should become part of your daily practice.

# 41. Technopathic Stress

With technopathic stress, the aim is blessing and harmonising the energies.

For individual pieces of equipment, e.g. Smart phone:

**Step 1:** Make sure that your psychic protection is in place.

**Step 2:** I like to hold the mobile phone between my hands and imagine a beam of white healing light entering it from above me, and as this happens, I recite the follow invocation:

**'To the Highest of the High I ask that all detrimental external and internal electro-magnetic energies in this smart phone be removed, taken to the light and disposed of appropriately.'**

**Step 3:** Then say:

**'I ask that the mobile phone be flooded with light and love, leaving it in peace, balance and harmony for family, friends, and animals.'**

**Step 4:** You can now repeat this for all devices in your home and workplace by reciting the following invocation (you do not have to have them between your hand, only the smaller objects):

**'To the Highest of the High I ask that all detrimental and inappropriate energy patterns are removed from (affected object) and taken to the light to be disposed of appropriately. I also ask that the (affected**

object) be flooded with light and love, leaving it in peace, balance and harmony for family, friends, and animals.'

**Step 5:** I carry out this procedure for the rest of the house including the wiring, Wi-Fi, 4G etc.

**'To the Highest of the High I ask that all external and internal electrical and electro-magnetic energies including Wi-Fi, in the home (or individual piece of equipment) be healed and that any and all detrimental energies be taken away and disposed of appropriately. I also ask that everything possible is done to harmonize the remaining energy patterns and frequencies, leaving them in peace, balance and harmony for family, friends, and animals. I ask that the healing takes place not only in this dimension but all other dimensions that are similarly affected.'**

*Step 6:* You can now dowse each device making sure it is no longer detrimental to the family or pets.

Some people are more sensitive than others to the effects of EMF's and they may not fully respond to this type of healing, especially if they are unwell or already suffering from a heavy dose of dirty electricity. Therefore, you may have to use one or more of the many scientific devices available to help further block or shield you from these rogue EMF's.

Alasdair Philips' website www.powerwatch.org.uk is worth visiting, as is the related www.emfields.org.

There is much research on the internet about the detrimental effect of cooking with microwave ovens, also the effect of long-life light bulbs on humans and animals. Please try and help yourself where you can, minimize your usage of mobile phones, change to the new LED-type bulbs that give off a healthy light and cook naturally.

Research is the key.

# 42. Human Interference Lines

**Step 1:** Check your psychic protection.

**Step 2:** Generally, it is a case of healing the line or lines with light and love, removing all the detrimental energy patterns and sending them to the light. Recite the following:

**'To the Highest of the High, I ask that the interference line (or lines) is being flooded with light and love, and as they are, all the detrimental thoughts, emotions and energies from it (them) are being removed and disposed of appropriately into the light'.**

**Step 3:** Flood the line (or lines) once again with light and love asking that they be left in peace, balance and harmony for all living things for all time.

**Step 4:** We also need to clear the detrimental effects of the interference line from the people it has affected. For this I would use the spiritual wall, placing each affected member of the family in their own individual rooms, and as they walk through the holy wall you recite the following:

**'To the Highest of the High, I ask that as (names) walk through the spiritual wall that their auras and physical bodies are cleared of all the detrimental energy caused by these man-made interference lines, and all that has been dislodged to be taken to the light and disposed of appropriately. I ask that the healing takes place not only in this dimension but all other dimensions that are similarly affected.'**

**Step 5:** We now place each member of the family in a bubble of white light that is mirrored on the outside, reflecting any further detrimental energy that might come their way.

**Step 6:** I also ask that these harmful energies are sent directly back to the source, to clear/heal whatever is responsible for setting up these interference lines including any humans that have been involved in the process. These are returned to the sender with unconditional love, as always, by reciting the following:

**'To the Highest of the High, please flood this line (lines) with healing light and love, sending it directly to those responsible for creating the detrimental energies, both to the humans involved and the machine itself. As these energy patterns are cleared, please take them to the light and dispose of them appropriately. I ask that the healing takes place not only in this dimension but all other dimensions that are similarly affected.'**

42

**Step 7:** Dowse to check that the lines are now cleared and are no longer detrimental to the family or home.

# 43. Fracture Lines Caused by Fracking

**Step 1:** Ensure your psychic protection is in place.

**Step 2:** Send healing to where the fracking is taking place by reciting the following:

**'To the Highest of the High, I ask that the fracking site now be flooded with light and love, and that all detrimental energies found there are taken away and disposed of appropriately into the light, leaving the area in peace, balance and harmony.'**

**Step 3:** Send healing to the workforce involved, continuing all the way up to senior level, by reciting the following:

**'To the Highest of the High, I ask that all persons involved in the fracking process, from the workers to the CEOs, have an ultra-fine mesh net of light and love pulled through their aura and physical body, removing all detrimental energy patterns and attachments, allowing them to see how they are desecrating our precious planet.'**

**Step 4:** Recite the following invocation to bring healing to the family and home:

**'To the Highest of the High, I ask that the fracking line affecting the family and their home is also flooded with light and love along its entire length, breadth and depth removing all detrimental energy patterns found within it, then to be taken to the light and disposed**

of in an appropriate fashion, leaving all lines in peace, balance and harmony for all living things for all time. I ask that the healing takes place not only in this dimension but all other dimensions that are similarly affected.'

**Step 5:** Dowse to check that the fracture lines are now clear of detrimental energies.

**NB** A lot of damage and fractures were also caused when the initial testing was being carried out, to see whether fracking was a viable option. These also need to be worked on and healing sent. Dowsing will help to show you whether you or your home has been affected or not.

43

# 44. Harmful Frequencies

To heal the harmful frequencies, carry out the following:

**Step 1:** Check that your psychic protection is in place.

**Step 2:** Recite the following:

**'To the Highest of the High, I wish to work on the detrimental frequencies, sounds and noises that are coming into my home from ......... Please send the necessary inverted healing sound to counteract and cancel the harmful sounds. Please remove all the detrimental energetic patterns, sending them to the light. Flood the sound waves with light and love leaving them in peace, balance and harmony.'**

**Step 3:** Dowse to check if the detrimental energies from these sounds are now clear.

# 45. Guardian of the Site, Spirit of Place or Home

**Step 1:** Make sure that your psychic protection is in place.

**Step 2:** Start a conversation with the guardian of the site, the spirit of place, or spirit of home (depending on which one is disgruntled) and find out why they are unhappy. Their issues can range from someone not tending their garden to a housing estate being built on their patch, formally a field or meadow.

**Step 3:** Ask them what you can do to make them happy. Sometimes, you can purely offer up an explanation of our modern lifestyle and that is all it takes. Perhaps they want you to plant a tree, for you to introduce certain colours in the home, even to perhaps bury crystals in the garden. You can receive their reply through dowsing, or meditation. Go with what thoughts come to your mind and be open to signs over the next few days.

**Step 4:** Send healing to them in the form of a rainbow asking that they be flooded with these beautiful colours and that any animosity they may feel be taken away and disposed of appropriately, so that they harmonize their energies with ours and help us with our lives.

**Step 5:** From now on, talk to the guardians/spirits, inform them what you are doing and why you are doing it, cutting down or pruning a tree for instance, why you are building an extension to your home, and, importantly introducing yourself to them, they like to know who you are.

Any house and earth energy healing that you are carrying out should put you into their good books, they like people who take care of the planet.

45

# 46. Elementals in the House and Detrimental Pathways

**Step 1:** Check that your psychic protection is in place.

**Step 2:** Call upon Uriel (the Archangel of the Earth) to assist you and recite the following:

'**Archangel Uriel, please pull an ultra-fine mesh net of light and love through the house and everyone in it, to gently gather up any elementals or nature spirits, wherever they may be, that are trapped or hiding. Placing them back into their natural habitat, asking them to care for and look after all the flora and fauna that they see.**'

**Step 3:** Speak to the elementals and explain why they have been moved. Ask them to dedicate themselves to the countryside around them, to look after the flora and fauna found locally, to be at peace in their new surroundings and to go with grace.

**Step 4:** Some elementals can be quite spiteful, causing your pets problems when they are out in the garden, if this is the case you can ask Archangel Uriel to remove all the detrimental and inappropriate nature spirits, placing them back into their natural countryside surroundings. Ask that they dedicate themselves to the local flora and fauna, going with grace.

## Nature spirit pathway:

**Step 1:** Make sure that your psychic protection is in place.

**Step 2:** We need to appease the local elementals, whatever they may be, due to someone or something blocking or disrupting their natural pathway. We do this by calling on Archangel Uriel once again and reciting the following:

'**Archangel Uriel, I call upon you to help appease the local nature spirits at (name of house). Sending healing to them and asking their forgiveness for us having disrupted their natural pathway by building an extension to our house (or whatever reason is, that caused the problem)'.**

**Step 3:** Then recite the following:

'**Archangel Uriel I now ask for you to clear any detrimental thoughts and actions, from the nature spirits, that may have caused us harm, for those patterns to be taken and disposed of appropriately into the earth, to leave our home and pathway in peace, balance and harmony for all living things. I ask that the healing takes place not only in this dimension but all other dimensions that are similarly affected.'**

**Step 4:** Finally recite out loud:

'**I ask that the disrupted pathway is now diverted, physically and energetically, from our home and any other property that has interrupted or blocked its natural direction. For it to now run harmlessly and undisturbed along the full extent of journey, sending peace and love to all the elementals that had been affected.'**

## Clearing ingested elementals:

**Step 1:** Ensure your psychic protection is in place.

**Step 2:** I would utilise the spiritual wall for this exercise, place the affected party in the spiritual waiting room, see them sitting in a chair until you are ready to move them through the holy wall. Now guide them through, their auric field first, and then their physical body, reciting the following:

'**To the Highest of the High, I ask that as (name) walks through the** spiritual wall that all the detrimental and inappropriate elementals that they may have ingested and are located in either their physical body or aura are being now being gently removed. When done, I ask that they are helped back into nature and once there, dedicate themselves to the wellbeing of the flora and fauna'.

**Step 3:** Finish with:

'I now send healing to those involved, leaving them all in peace, balance and harmony'.

46

# 47. Tree Spirits

**Step 1:** Ensure your psychic protection is in place.

**Step 2:** If you have found a suitable tree or shrub in the garden, that does not already have its own tree spirit, simply ask Archangel Uriel to relocate the displaced tree spirit, asking it to dedicate itself to the tree's wellbeing, now and in the future.

**Step 3:** If you have not found a suitable tree you may need to buy one for your garden. When it has been planted, simply ask Uriel's assistance in helping the displaced tree spirit move. Ask it to dedicate its life to the wellbeing and growth of the newly planted shrub or tree.

You can also hold a short dedication ceremony if you wish, without invoking Archangel Uriel. A few kind words spoken out loud, introducing the tree to the misplaced spirit, and asking it to move across and link itself to your new purchase, then dedicating itself to the trees wellbeing and sturdy growth.

**Step 4:** Placing a crystal beneath the tree as you plant it can help transmute any detrimental energy lines that might affect its growth. Dowse to see if a) A crystal would be beneficial for it safety and growth and b) what crystal or crystals it should be.

**Step 5:** In a few weeks you can dowse to make sure that all is well and both tree and its incumbent spirit are happy.

# 48. Animal Spirits

**Step 1:** Dowse to ensure your psychic protection is in place.

**Step 2:** Recite the following invocation:

**'To the Highest of the High, please shine a beam of beautiful light in front of each lost soul and show each of them a vision of what awaits them in Heaven. Their own idea of perfection.'**

**Step 3:** Speak directly to the animal spirits, reciting the following animal spirit release invocation:

48

**'Please do not be afraid by this form of communication as I have been granted special dispensation to talk to you today, to help you to continue your interrupted journey into the light. I have asked that your owner (if already passed away) or your parents be with you now, to assist and guide you on your journey.**

**I have asked Archangel Zadkiel to cut any cords that have held you back from naturally going to the light and cleared away any attachments and I now, therefore invite you to move into the light, and to be with your family once again. Amen.'**

**Step 4:** After waiting a few minutes, dowse to make sure that all the souls have gone to the light. Then enquire if there are any further lost souls that wish to go to the light today. Remember the layer system; it might be that the lead spirit has now gone, freeing up others to move through.

Check for a third time, to be on the safe side – asking 'do I need to move any further spirits through today?'

**Step 5:** Say out loud:

**'Highest of the High, please send my love to all the souls who have now moved into the light, ensuring that they are now happy. I also ask that any doorways, opened expectedly or unexpectedly during my dowsing/healing work, are now firmly closed, that any residue left behind by the lost souls passing through is removed and taken into the light, leaving the house in peace, balance and harmony. I ask that the healing takes place not only in this dimension but all other dimensions that are similarly affected.'**

Once they have successfully moved through, they can return at any stage to be with their family and also to help you with your healing sessions.

# 49. Animal Created Stress Lines

To clear and heal these lines, you may need to work on the pets and their owners, any farm animals (cows, sheep, pigs, chickens etc.) and the farmers. All the mental and physical anguish needs to be addressed and dealt with.

**Step 1:** Make sure that your psychic protection is in place.

**Step 2:** Recite the following:

'**To Archangel Uriel, I ask that all detrimental energy patterns created by any physical and mental cruelty to animals are now cleared from these lines, taken to the light and disposed of correctly. Please flood the stress with light and love leaving them in peace, balance and harmony.**'

**Step 3:** Using the Spiritual Wall method, visualise the farmers, pet owners, breeders, or kennel owners and helpers moving from the spiritual waiting room, through the holy wall into the divine white light room, while repeating the following invocation:

'**To Archangel Uriel, as these people move through the holy wall, I ask they are being cleared of any detrimental or inappropriate attachments, or energies that have caused them (knowingly or unknowingly) to harm animals, whether mentally or physically. I ask that any energies left behind in the spiritual waiting room are now taken into the light and disposed of appropriately. I ask that** the healing takes place not only in this dimension but all other dimensions that are similarly affected.'

**Step 4:** Flood the line with light and love, asking for it to be left in peace, balance and harmony for humans and animals. I then suggest that you check to see that it is no longer detrimental.

The places where these lines have originated, such as boarding kennels, stables or people's houses, may need regularly work because even though you have carried out a healing, new animals and pets could arrive at any time necessitating further healing to be done.

It is also a good idea to carry out a clearing/healing of any pet that may have been in kennels for any length of time as they too can pick up attachments, both from humans and elementals. You can use the spiritual wall or the ultra-fine mesh net of light and love to clear them.

Make sure that you do this before you bring them home, so that you have not allowed any nasties to follow them home.

49

# 50. Any beneficial areas to sit/meditate

This is the only completely positive question that I ask. Everything else that we do is purely to find the detrimental energies that have impacted us and our families and deal with them.

It may be that you are lucky enough to have one of these 'energetic areas' naturally occurring in your home, but if not then we need to go about creating one. This will allow you to sit, utilise and absorb the beneficial healing power of the earth.

Intention is the key and meditation will help you achieve it.

**Step 1:** Pick a location in your home where you would like this special area to be, ideally in a room where you can sit quietly and just be.

**Step 2:** As you start to meditate your intention is to build up a positive energy or a higher vibration, this will start to attract beneficial energy lines to your location, eventually they will cross but this will be down to repetition.

**Step 3:** Try to meditate on that spot every day, at the same time for a few weeks, setting the same intention.

As you read in the chapter on energy channels, many of the earth's energies will react to human consciousness and by engaging with them regularly, you will find that they will be attracted to your spiritual intention and move, creating a healing space.

50

**Step 4:** Once the lines have crossed and you have created your beneficial/healing area, ask Upstairs to anchor it in place. Then whenever you need to do any healing on yourself or family, this will be the place to sit

# 51. Energising/Healing Rays

**Step 1:** Ensure your psychic protection is in place.

**Step 2:** This is all about you, bathing yourself in your chosen colour (or the colour you dowsed that is needed). Dowse to find out how long you need to sit for and, what time is the most beneficial for you to do so. Colour is good for you, it energises the mind, body and soul, as well as boosting and strengthening your aura.

**Step 3:** Sit quietly and visualise (or just ask for, if you find visualisation difficult) a beam of coloured light coming from above, enveloping you, bringing you healing, love and wellness.

**Step 4:** Once the time is up, you can dowse to find out how beneficial this colour shower has been, start counting slowly from 1 to 10 and wait for the rod or pendulum to move, the nearer to 10 it gets, the more beneficial it has been.

51

# 52. Anything else to be considered regarding the health of the people

There is no healing to be done in this section, necessarily, but you may find that you will need a particular flower remedy to help balance your mind and body, and those of your family, whilst you undergo the changes brought about by the clearing/healing process you have just gone through.

Healing will bring big changes into your life. They can be very subtle to begin with, but they will happen. Ridding or clearing your mind of all the pent up and stored emotional energies from the past means that new energy patterns can come in, helping you to see more clearly and then move forwards in many different ways.

It is good to soften the landing if possible, and a short course of flower remedies can help you and the family have that. Dowsing will help you choose the right one, work out how many drops you need, when to take them and how long for.

You can also dowse a whole range of vitamins and supplements working out which are best for you and your family but if in doubt please consult a good naturopath or homeopath.

You can also dowse for food intolerances and allergies, general health issues; and you can compile your own list or download any of the following from my online store at: www.dowsingspirits.co.uk.

Australian Bush Flower Remedies

Bach Flower Remedies

Food Allergy Checklist

Household and Environmental Chart

How to remain grounded

Psychic Protection

Questions to ask at Sacred Sites

Who is my Spirit Guide?

Who is my Animal Guide?

How to Dowse

52

# 53. Is there anything else that is detrimental for me to find?

Depending on the answer you receive to this question, you may need to employ several of the healing methods in this to clear anything that you may have found. This is where you get to adapt the methods that I have described in this book and match them to the specific issue or issues that have emerged.

Just remember to make sure that your psychic protection is fully in place, and once the problem has been cleared or healed, you ask that any doors that have been opened expectedly or unexpectedly are firmly closed.

If you cannot work out what the issues is, or are stuck on how to heal it, I am more than happy to receive an email from you, (adrian@ dowsingspirits.co.uk) and will assist you as best as I can.

53

# 54. Family DNA clearing and Healing

**Step 1:** Ensure that your psychic protection is in place.

**Step 2:** Simply visualise your paternal and maternal ancestral family lines stretching before you, it looks rather like a spider's web as there are many strands, going back generations. Channel the healing light from above (via your crown chakra) moving it down to your heart chakra then push it out, watching it travel along the complex network of your ancestral pathways.

**Step 3:** During this visualisation, recite the following:

**'To the Highest of the High, I send this healing light along my ancestral pathway asking that it clear away any detrimental and inappropriate energy patterns coming from my forebears, including any attachments, curses, miasms and diseases that may have travelled the family lines as well as clearing away any detrimental energies contained within their DNA strands. As these energetic patterns are removed, they are to be taken into the Universe and disposed of in the correct fashion. I send my love, understanding and gratitude to all of my relatives, leaving the family line in peace, balance and harmony for all time. I ask that the healing takes place not only in this dimension but all other dimensions that are similarly affected.'**

**Step 4:** Dowse to check that your DNA is healed of all past illnesses and diseases, and then ask if there is anything further you need to do. An

54

ancestor may need moving to the light or forgiveness sent to one or more of your forebears.

**Step 5:** Finally recite the following:

**'To the Highest of the High I ask for any doorways that have been opened expectedly or unexpectedly during the course of my dowsing/ healing work are now firmly closed, that any residue left behind by lost souls passing through is also removed and taken into the light, leaving the family and house in peace, balance and harmony.'**

**Step 6:** Dowse to check if the DNA is now clear and if there are any more layers that have been revealed that need healing.

# Closing Down

This is very important part of the healing process.

Just as we have an opening ritual linking us to the Universe, Mother Earth, Our Life-Giving Sun and Heavenly Moon, when we have finished our healing work, we need to have a closing down ceremony; not just to give thanks to those who have been working with us, but also to return our heightened energetic state to normal living levels.

I see it as a way of closing and then locking the office door, it signifies the end to your working day, allowing you to return to the physical life on Earth.

It is a simple Invocation:

**'To the Highest of the High, Mother Earth, our Life-Giving Sun and Heavenly Moon thank you for using me as your healing instrument here on the planet.**

**I would ask that any doorways or portals that were opened expectedly or unexpectedly, in this and any other dimension, during the course of my healing work are now firmly closed.**

**I would like to thank all the Archangels and Angels that have been with me, all spirits, my spirit guides, healing guides and protection guides, I ask that I am now fully grounded and that my energies return to normal living levels. Amen.'**

I would suggest that you work on your own home before attempting to work on someone else's property. As you experience the changes, be aware and make note of how your mind, body and soul feel, how your sleep patterns change, how the family dynamics alter, the general atmosphere of the house and so on.

# The Settling Down Period

Once complete, it is now important to let the healing sink in.

Make sure that psychically protect yourself every morning. Do not forget that you can also include each member of your family as you sit and psychically protect yourself.

Some clients will feel the impact immediately, but for most families the effects tend to be phased in, thereby avoiding the roller coaster ride that can follow a big emotional release or potentially prompt a 'Healing Crisis'.

By using the word 'appropriate' in our healing, it sends a message to Upstairs to send healing to each member of the family when the time is right for them. I see healers rather like the conductor of an orchestra, each member is an expert musician, but you need an outside individual to bring everything together in a cohesive manner.

All we can control is how and when we carry out the detective work and the healing. The Higher Realms know so much more about the timings than we do, they will send the necessary healing when it is the correct time to do so.

Once the initial healing phase has settled in (around two weeks), I like to check to make sure that all is well, sometimes layers appear and need to be dealt with as they emerge. Therefore, feedback from the family is important. So, set yourself a reminder, for about ten to fourteen days after the initial healing has taken place, to take stock of new energy levels, any illnesses (flu like symptoms for example) and how the home feels. Then dowse the checklist again to see if there are any more layers that have risen to the surface and can now be dealt with.

Also make a note in your diary or set a reminder, to go through the checklist every two months to start with, and then as reoccurrences lessen, every six months. But do try to implement the psychic protection method on a regular basis, ideally every morning, and if you can, encourage your family to do so as well. This will lessen the likelihood of nasties entering the home even more.

When my boys were younger, at school and then college, I would check them most days for attachments and carry out a clearing. You would be surprised how many they would pick up during the day. So, I would recommend a regular clearing of your children, as they return home from school, before they come into the house.

# Healing Effects

Clients have reported bright lights appearing in their home shortly after the healing has taken place, others feel that the house feels warmer and brighter, one lady said that her house seemed less fuzzy, that all the rooms and furniture now had a clarity to them that wasn't there before.

In a few cases, my clients have reported that, after I have carried out my healing, there has been no changes in either the family or house, nothing appears to have happened. My first thought is that I have lost it, that Upstairs have cast me adrift, or taken away my ability to help others. Those doubts normally last for a few moments before I pick up my pendulum and ask the question 'Is this truly the case', and I have always got a 'no' response. Something has happened, but as yet it is too subtle for the family to notice. I then breathe a sigh of relief.

It is purely down to timing, so hold the intention that the healing has been done correctly and check for any layers and deal with them as required. Accept that fine-tuning the healing can take days, weeks and sometimes months. It really does depend on how deep the problems were in the first place as it may have taken many years for the home to become so detrimental, therefore healing the family and their home is rarely something that can be completed in a day or two.

So do take your time, expect the unexpected and enjoy the ride.

# Afterword

It is said that everyone has a book inside them, but I admit to never feeling this way, in fact I was told by my English teacher at my Secondary school in Suffolk that I would never be able to write one.

Looking back, I have always been prone to dyslexia, not as bad as some but certainly enough to find writing difficult, until I discovered the computer keyboard (and spell checker, although that can easily add to my confusion). It helps slow my mind down, having to concentrate on which key to press.

Writing with a pen allows my brain to work faster than my hand, and the resulting mess (or words) resembles shorthand, and sometimes even I can't read what I have put down on paper. So, the keyboard is paramount to you being able to read this book and hopefully understand it.

I tend not to suffer from writer's block because of the way that I write. A good friend and author of several recommended dowsing books, Nigel Twinn, said 'Adrian I would find it very difficult to edit your book; you write as though you are talking to someone sitting in front of you and that is very different to what I do'.

Michelle Gordon, my editor and also the editor to a number of other lucky people, helped me pull my first book together, taking out countless exclamation marks (several hundred I believe), proof reading, taking out even more exclamation marks and some inflammatory comments (my parental patterning), then using the checklist to work on and heal her Mother's home.

Sally Byrne, Michelle's mum, helped massively too, she looked at what I had written from a completely different perspective. It was all well and good me understanding what I had written, but I needed to make sure that it was comprehensible and usable from a non-dowser's point of view, even though Sally is very spiritually minded.

This book is as comprehensive as I can make it today. I have no doubt that other problems will present themselves as we move through the 21st century: new inventions will bring new energies that will need to be dealt with in new ways. As we all become more sensitive, as seems to be the case, the more people will need the help of Earth Healers (Geomancers) and Home Healers to allow them to lead a peaceful, healthy lifestyle, living in harmony, not just with themselves, but also with Mother Nature.

I hope that you have found this book useful in clearing and healing yourself, your family and home.

By logging on to my website and leaving your name and email address I can keep you fully up to date with courses and future publications.

Website: www.dowsingspirits.co.uk

Email: adrian@dowsingspirits.co.uk

# About Adrian

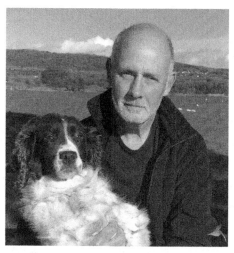

Dowsing has featured in Adrian's life since he was seven, but it never dawned on him that it would have such an impact on him later in his life.

Owning a busy Estate Agency in Surrey inspired him to look at the repeating patterns of divorce in certain homes, and from that Dowsing Spirits was born. To help people be healthy and happy and have harmonious relationships, Adrian checks for detrimental energies in people and their homes, and then heals them. His clients have included several royal families, a number of well-known film stars and many successful businesses throughout the world.

For three years, he was the Vice President of the British Society of Dowsers and was chair of both their Earth Energies and Health dowsing groups.

His self-help book, *Heal Your Home*, has been described as the bible of geopathic stress and has a worldwide readership. He also wrote 'Spirit & Earth with Tim Walter. One of his missions in life is to bring dowsing into the 21st century and is fulfilling this by teaching various courses and giving talks around the UK and Europe.

He lives with his wife, Allyson, and springer spaniel, Annie, in a small village near Richmond in the Yorkshire Dales.

## Also available from Adrian:

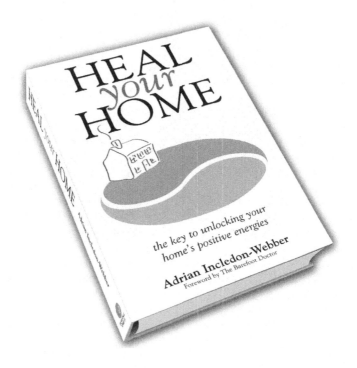

# Heal Your Home

Often referred to as 'the bible of geopathic stress' this best-selling book is the 'go-to' for anyone interested in, not just earth energies but many other noxious problems that affect their home, office or workspace. The book describes, in down to earth terms, how to locate and then deal with the detrimental energies that can affect us in our daily lives, including spirits, earth energy lines, inherited human emotions, attachments, psychic attack, curses and much more. Importantly it has been written as a self-help book with a detailed section on how to carry out a healing yourself.

Get your copy now from www.dowsingspirits.co.uk

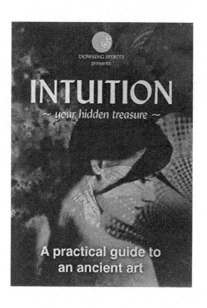

# Intuition – Your Hidden Treasure

This DVD is a treasure house of information on how to develop your sixth sense through dowsing. Many subjects are covered from how to make and use dowsing rods, what to look for at ancient sites, working how detrimental your household products can be, horse racing, how psychic protection helps a rock band, how vibrations can help enliven sacred sites and more.

Get your copy now from www.dowsingspirits.co.uk

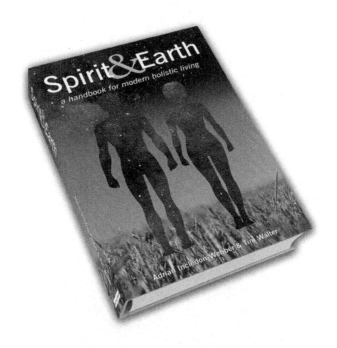

# Spirit & Earth

With the exception of Feng Shui, 'House Healing' is not a widely accepted practice. This book has been written by two of the world's most eminent practitioners in what has become known as modern Geomancy. Working with subtleties that can be accessed through meditation, mindfulness and dowsing this book shows how the power of focused intent can be harnessed to improve the relationship between humans, buildings, nature and Mother Earth in simple, practical ways. The authors have spent decades helping people subtly change the way they function in their homes and here they share their experience, knowledge and philosophy to illustrate how, by changing the perceptions of our lives through truly holistic thinking, we can create a sustained positive relationship with everything around us.

Get your copy now from www.dowsingspirits.co.uk

## *If you would like to get in touch*

You can follow Adrian on the usual social media platforms or email him directly:

Email: adrian@dowsingspirits.co.uk

Website: www.dowsingspirits.co.uk

The website gives up-to-date information and details on workshops and dowsing courses which include:

The Secrets of Healing Your Home I, II and III
Introduction to Dowsing
Dowsing for Health I and II
Earth Energies I
Healing with Sacred Symbols
Spirit & Earth I, II and III


## *Independent Publishing Services were provided by:*

The Amethyst Angel
theamethystangel@hotmail.co.uk
NotFromThisPlanet.co.uk

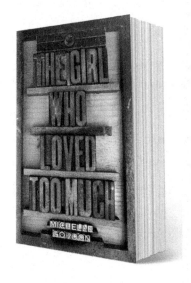
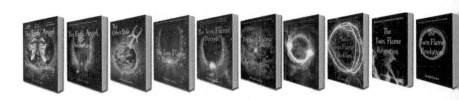

Made in the USA
Coppell, TX
20 May 2021